A DOCTOR'S REFLECTIONS ON CHANGE

The Natural World, Farming,

Medicine, Travel and Global Health

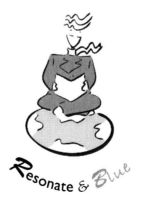

Resonate & Blue

First published by **Resonate** & *Blue* in 2016

(Imprint of **Tatterdemalion** *Blue*)

Words © Eric Walker 2016

Photographs © Eric Walker 2016

A CIP catalogue record for this book
is available from the British Library

Cover design and layout by **Tatterdemalion** *Blue*

ISBN 978-0-9933114-4-4

Tatterdemalion *Blue*
21 Underwood Cottages
Cambusbarron
Stirling
FK7 9PA

www.tatterdemalionblue.com

A Doctor's Reflections on Change

The Natural World, Farming,

Medicine, Travel and Global Health

7/7/16

Dear Lucia
I thought you might
enjoy some of these historical memories
especially the ones on the evolution
of travel and global health
Best wishes and love
Eric

Eric Walker

CONTENTS

Acknowledgements

This little book would not have ever begun without the original suggestion and continual encouragement of Kerryann Cope, a close friend and nursing colleague.

I am especially grateful to my long-standing friend and travel medicine colleague Robert Steffen for writing an introductory preface and for his helpful and kind contribution.

I thank Pip Ryan for checking over the proofs. Leslie Mair for help preparing the illustration for the front cover and importantly John King who, as my publisher, has given me as a novice writer personal guidance, as well as other friends and family members who have made helpful suggestions along the way.

The cover illustration

The Scottish mountains can be seen to reflect prehistoric times and adventure. The sight and sounds of flowing water reminds us that life's journey is constantly changing. The small images symbolize how cultural and time differences influence how we work with our natural surroundings.

PREFACE

You are holding in your hands a precious account of an interesting life. Eric Walker like many others boys born during World War II constructed Spitfire models, got lost in the fog as a scout and was excited about the first car of his parents. But already in childhood he was an exceptional kid with broader interests. He then started to keep honeybees and he won an early prize for 'six brown eggs' as a very young chicken and rabbit farmer. Despite his great interest in nature and the environment he abandoned this career to study medicine.

These memoirs are fascinating in many ways. For the older generation, they revive memories long lost. To the young readership they illustrate how dramatically different life was up to some seventy years ago. Then there were not even visions or dreams about things like mobile phones - the switchboards to connect a call then were still being used and not exhibited in museums. Particularly for medical professionals it is instructive to be reminded of infectious diseases in the pre-antibiotic area. That also was a period in which hardly any vaccines had been developed.

The author gained a broad personal and professional experience during his stays abroad, especially during prolonged and multiple working periods in India. That and his genuine diagnostic skills made him a highly esteemed leader in infectious and tropical diseases as well as in public health both there and back home. Many far beyond Scotland of course remember how Eric was among the first globally to see a need to develop travel medicine both by offering advice to future travellers and by conducting successful research together with a group of colleagues. A lecturer initially in India, later in Glasgow, he played an increasingly leading role in medical education culminating in being the Dean of the new Faculty of Travel Medicine - the only of its kind worldwide.

Rather than adhering to the profit orientated approach in modern medicine he throughout his entire career with highest ethical standards kept in mind the underprivileged in India and elsewhere. Luxury travel health was not his priority but to contribute to the well-being of those in greatest need. Compassion and empathy are the traits of his noble character - and that makes this autobiography truly valuable.

Having read this book, many like myself will lean back and be a little jealous wondering: why did I not take notes starting as a youngster, maintain a diary?

Thank you Eric for having offered this insight into your life - our lifetime - now the lifetime of grandparents.

Zurich, 22 March 2016

Robert Steffen

A Doctor's Reflections on Change

on Change

The Natural World, Farming,

Medicine, Travel and Global Health

INTRODUCTION

Having grown up at a time when 'waste not, want not' and taking personal responsibility to avoid health risks was normal practice, it is easy to see how many things have changed since the mid 20th century. For me, with a love of nature and the countryside from an early age and an appreciation of the importance of how human behaviour and our environment are inextricably bound together, this was accepted without question.

Both my farming experience and medicine involve caring effectively for the environment, for animals, plants and fellow human beings; involving similar prevention, diagnostic and management approaches. An interest in biology and infection has been a thread through all of this combined with early opportunities to travel and explore.

The changes in lifestyles and attitudes to the environment that have taken place over the last 100 years are enormous. The majority of us now live in cities, we are less aware of our dependent relationship with nature for food and health. Going to the countryside; looking out of car windows, stopping in a village for tea, chips or ice cream is now simply a form of weekend entertainment or tourism for many.

We have motorised vehicles which have progressively replaced walking, horses and horse drawn carriages, sailing ships, bicycles and towed barges as means of transport. Much of this has been a result of our enormous increase in knowledge gained through scientific research - for example, the widespread availability of combustion engines and electricity. However, there is a cost to this when it is very dependent 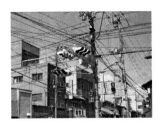 on finite energy resources such as coal, oil and gas.

We can now travel rapidly to virtually anywhere in the world and communicate digitally in real-time through mass media and individually. However, what are the effects on speech, face-to-face communication and body language?

Rather than fulfilling our basic human health needs, many of the changes are now motivated by commercial aspirations and we commonly prepare our children to work for others whose motivation is profit before service, rather than philanthropic tasks they personally believe in. As a result, in our 'developed' countries we have so many mass-produced goods and so much food available that we create huge amounts of waste. This rubbish is non-existent in the natural environment and the term itself is of recent origin. It is interesting to surmise what would happen if we ceased to have access to electricity. I have been involved recently in setting

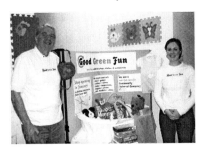 up a very successful local reusing/recycling charity shop 'Good Green Fun', which helps minimise the huge waste of children's clothes, toys, books, prams, games, cots etc.,

which so often are stored unused in attics, under beds or end up in landfill sites. I believe its success reflects the beginnings of a change in attitude to waste.

In modern life, our senses are overwhelmed by electronic images and sounds through television, advertising, computers, mobile phones and noisy transport. Yet how often do we reflect on the often quieter and subtler images and sounds of nature such as wildlife, the weather, our own breathing and conversations? We need to question if our basic needs have really changed significantly over time. Is it sustainable to use scientific knowledge, simply because it is there, without considering if the consequences may be more harmful than beneficial?

Recently however, there appears to be an increasing interest in some long-standing and well-tried-and-tested practices. In the food industry, for example, there seems to be a small, but real, reaction against mass-production, wastage, and putting profit before health. The phrase 'from the garden to the table' proposes that local sustainable fruit and vegetable growing can minimise costs and improve quality. The implementation can be a personal or a community endeavour.

To cope with this often-confusing mental merry-go-round some are now looking to more traditional techniques for coping with these stresses. For example, allocating time to focus on the 'here and now' can help us to more easily develop healthy relationships with others and with our environment. But this is not easy since it is not common practice and requires adjustment to our daily lifestyles.

The many and varied techniques include deep relaxation through focused breathing, self-hypnosis, meditation, yoga, controlling our thoughts through 'mindfulness', and the recognition of transience. All of these throughout history have been embedded in peace seeking and love focused religions.

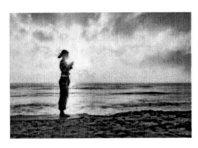

No doubt we will see many lifestyles and environmental changes in the future and the 'doctor's journey' will continue ...

Early Childhood in Birmingham

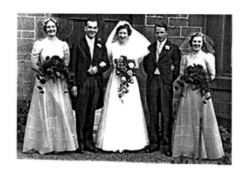

My parents migrated from Scotland to England in the 1930s when my father set up a dental practice in Birmingham and was appointed as consultant in dental surgery at the new Queen Elizabeth Hospital. He had previously worked in a dental practice in Elgin. They had grown up and met in Edinburgh when at university. As well as being qualified in dentistry, my father trained in medicine which was, and still is, a requirement to practice facio-maxillary surgery. As his parents were not able to pay the necessary fees, he was only able to enter Edinburgh University through gaining scholarships, as state-funding was not available at that time. My mother studied and qualified as a chartered accountant, and used these skills to help my father run his dental practice and act as treasurer for many charities and voluntary organisations. She could add up long lists of pounds, shillings and pence in her head (not many of us can do that these days!).

My paternal grandfather was a primary school head teacher in Dalmeny, which is close to the famous Forth Bridge near Edinburgh, and he died around the time my father went to university, when in his 40s, from rheumatic heart disease. My maternal grandfather grew up in Bo'ness. He was a school teacher and later became rector (headmaster) of Lindsey Academy in Bathgate. As was usual in those days, both my grandmothers gave up employment (teaching and work in the post office respectively) soon after they were married.

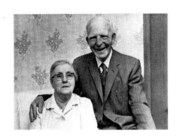

I got to know my maternal grandparents best since, during early childhood days, holidays were spent regularly with them in Ayr. Much time was spent on the beach. My grandmother was one of the very first people to have a full hip replacement following a fracture. Unfortunately, it soon slipped out of place but she declined further surgery, and for the rest of her life had a limp. She needed a stick for support for as long as I knew her.

The improvement in healthcare facilities since the 19th and early 20th centuries is dramatically illustrated by the reduction in childhood deaths, and both my grand-parents had several siblings who did not reach their teens. Mostly due to respiratory spread infections such as tuber-culosis, diphtheria and scarlet fever, closely followed by childhood diarrhoeal illnesses, typhoid and cholera.

Early Post-World War II Experiences

In some ways it feels a bit surreal to describe this period. I was born at home in the middle of World War II in 1943 in Kings Norton, a village close to Birmingham that has since become a suburb. Contributing to this separation from reality was that, as noted by many historians, war experiences were rarely mentioned or discussed later 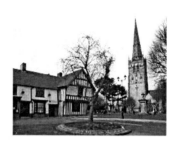 by those directly involved. This included my parents and the memories were clearly too painful to talk about freely. Maybe this reluctance to discuss the issues openly is a reason why many of us still are aware of reflex apprehension when we meet people from or visit the countries with which we were at war. After the War, everyone was focused on rebuilding their lives and careers, and for some this meant finding new homes. A government initiative was to build large numbers of standard 'prefabs' which were like static versions of the mobile homes of today. Most residents of these small houses took a great pride in keeping them attractive and well maintained.

Our understanding of events, even years later, is still regularly reawakened by historical archives on television and semi-fictional war films whose role at the time was mainly to boost morale. I was one of those who made up detailed and very realistic models of Spitfire, Hurricane and Lancaster airplanes from kits - perhaps fewer would have been made if children then had access to television and computers instead of enjoying handcrafts!

I was too young when living in Kings Norton to have verbal memories but I visually recollect blackout curtains which had to be carefully drawn each evening, the bomb-shelter at the foot of the garden and being gazed at in my cot by 'an owl'. This was probably my Auntie Elizabeth, lovingly checking up on me, with her large, round spectacles. I cannot confirm its validity, but I have an image in my mind of being taken across the street by my mother after a bombing raid, and seeing from the street, one of the occupants sitting up dazed in his bath. The front wall of the house had been destroyed. Rosebay willow herb was in abundance since its feathery seeds made it the first flowering plant to establish itself on bomb-sites. I now see it mainly as an important source of nectar for my honeybees.

For many years afterwards, well into my teens, I used to have nightmares of armies marching up our driveway that sometimes led me to cry out and hide under my bed to be rescued by my concerned mother. It is difficult to understand the significance of these 'playbacks'. However, many of us continued to have severe anxieties, sometimes irrational, about the inevitability of catastrophe whenever war or threat of wars have surfaced since. These apprehensions were fueled by the prolonged Cold War from the early 1960s, when countries set about developing arsenals of atom bombs and nuclear weapons. A big change now is that we have to adjust to international news arriving in real-time, electronically, so the truth about modern day threats and conflicts quickly comes in for worldwide public scrutiny. However, this real-time news is often undigested and can be initially inaccurate, which has to be taken into account. The days of news only by word of mouth, horseback, letters (snail mail) and daily newspapers have gone.

The stresses, anxieties and fears experienced in wartime must have had a considerable impact on those involved. In my parents' and grandparents' case perhaps even more so, since they had also witnessed the First World War. It is only in later life that I have become much more aware of how the War shaped the future for my parents and had an influence on children born around that period. While it was not something children at the time thought much about, the immediate recovery period and austerity after the War lasted at least 10-15 years and had a major affect on our early lives. Many of my generation enjoyed happy-ending films and books in our youth. This may well be due to the clearly defined and comforting difference they made between right and wrong. These were issues the War had left us confused about.

Many of us became suspicious of anything German or Japanese, and only later did some of us slowly realise that there is a difference between the world of international politics and the universal, and more simple, needs and as-pirations of individual people. It seems citizens can become insidiously, often unknowingly at the time, involved in awful behaviour and events where human life becomes cheap and expendable. We still see this happening in the 21st century in similar fashion to many of the horrors described in the Old Testament of the Bible. Sadly, little of these forms of human behaviour seem to change - just the methods and equipment used to wreak havoc and destruction. Due to the large number of men killed, I became aware of unmarried or widowed women. These were friends of my parents or family members and the real reason for their situation was never discussed.

Family and Friends

Deep family friendships were very important to us and I will describe one in particular, from my teenage years, with our farming neighbours. The word 'partners' did not exist although I was aware of some common-law informal marriages that could be considered to be the same thing.

I have an older brother and younger sister, but my parents had two other sons who died shortly after birth from cystic fibrosis, one just before I was born and one after. Around this time my father was posted abroad to India which must have put an enormous strain on my mother. I only found out about my deceased brothers by accident in my teens when I came across their birth certificates. This had never been mentioned previously and it was a bit of a shock and even on discovery was not discussed in any detail. These events contributed to the creation of a very close relationship between my family and our neighbours, Eric and Elizabeth Vincent, who had no children of their own.

They befriended my parents, particularly my mother in my father's absence.

My adopted Uncle Eric was managing director of a very successful factory making Blue Bird toffees and sweets, which his father had founded during the 19th century. Uncle Eric and Auntie Elizabeth were very 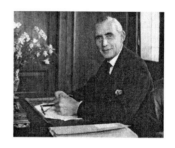 close and I understood that his family had disapproved of the marriage because she was his secretary and so he was considered to be marrying below his status. Although I cannot know for sure, I feel certain this friendship is how I happened to be called 'Eric', or at least, I like to think so. They had a lovely dog, with long droopy ears, who I adored.

The Blue Bird factory was a mini-Cadburys developed as an altruistic business where the workers were carefully and generously looked after with housing, stores, social support, pensions, recreation and sports facilities. Some now cynically call this approach to social care 'pater-nalistic', but that is certainly not how I saw it at the time and the factory workers I remember held my Uncle Eric in

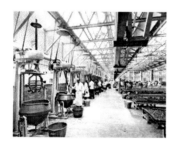 high regard. I joined in cricket matches with staff on their own cricket pitch, admired the ornate furnishings of the factory boardroom and vividly remember taking our paper bags, before the days of

plastic, into the factory at Christmas. We filled them up with sweets of our choice from the chutes before they tumbled into various sweet containers for distribution. Blue Bird was famous for its colourful 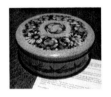 and attractively designed tins in which my Uncle Eric took a personal interest. Most of them had a special Blue Bird logo printed on them.

Our First House Move and Continuing Austerity

When I was aged 3 years we moved to Edgbaston (1946-50) nearer the centre of Birmingham. In addition to his job as a consultant facio-maxillary surgeon, my father ran a private dentistry practice from our house. This was still a time of severe austerity, although we did not call it such. Looking back it makes recent recessions seem insignificant, although a difference was that unemployment was less with all the building reconstruction that had to be carried out. Wages however, were proportionately very much lower and half-day Saturday working was normal. The consumer society had not yet arrived. Current efforts to discourage waste by refusing,

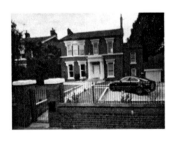 reusing and recycling were then normal practice. 'Waste not, want not' and 'clean up your plate' were slogans that everyone used. Rationing of meat, petrol, sugar and sweets continued well into the 1950s.

Some of our favourite foods were corned beef sandwiches, bread and butter pudding and french toast made with dried egg powder. Many years later we still had cans of wartime egg powder in the house, which I used to take on camping trips. They were perfectly useable 15 years later, there were no misleading use-by dates in those days.

Those, including my father, who established their own fruit and vegetable gardens to contribute to the war effort, kept these skills going after the War. I remember being chased all around the garden, screaming, by an aggressive bantam cockerel and learnt the hard way that bantams are renowned for protecting their harems vigorously. Their eggs were greatly appreciated, and I learnt how to place them in a bowl of water to check if they were still usable: floating meant they had gone bad. Hens running truly free-range lay fewer eggs during the winter, and if we had too many eggs during the summer they were put in a bucket of water containing 'water glass' (sodium silicate) which would preserve them by making the shells airtight.

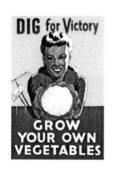

In winter we relied on several layers of clothing, warm gloves, and all-enclosing home-knitted balaclavas to keep warm. We used hot-water bottles and open coal, or bar electric fires. During very cold periods, mains water taps were turned off in the evening and the pipes drained to prevent the water inside freezing and bursting the pipes due to water expansion - one of our first physics lessons.

The only pipe insulation available was hessian, the same as used to make sacks, and we were very suspicious of plastic pipes and polystyrene which was, in any case, not easily available. Most mains water supplies passed through large tanks in house lofts for distribution through gravity feed. This allowed a store of water to be available when the mains supplies were unavailable. Sediments could settle on the bottom but they were also liable to freezing up.

A regular adventure was trips by bus to a large store in the centre of Birmingham. Downstairs was a barber's where hand-operated clippers were used to cut our hair. In the same department we bought new shoes, and our feet were always x-rayed to check the size was correct. This was not considered to be a health risk at the time and my feet still seem normal! At this time, 'luminous watches', where the numbers and hands had been touched-up with radioactive paint, were still common. The shop also had a fascinating system where money paid was whisked off in a special metal container through a suction tube to the store's central cash point, and change was sent back in similar fashion. We were sometimes allowed to load it up.

I must have been quite a shy infant because I remember going to a birthday party in the local botanical gardens and being terrified by the prospect of being the last person left on the floor during a game of musical chairs (winning the prize meant nothing). My mother had to be called in to take me home early because I was crying inconsolably. I have often since been wary of being in the spotlight especially in situations where I don't know quite what might happen. Maybe this is why I chose later to learn to play the viola since, unlike the violins, it meant I did not need to sit in the front rows of the orchestra!

As young children, we were encouraged to save some pocket money in National Savings Certificates. This was a new savings scheme to provide extra resources for the government. They are, of course, still available now sixty years later.

Teenage Years
in Rural Worcestershire

A Car Changed Our Lives

After 4 years in Edgbaston, when I was about 6 years old, my father acquired a car. Cars at this time were unusual. They all had starting handles so that the car could be started mechanically without using a battery driven starter motor. It was important to know how to hold the handle with your thumb tucked in above your fingers to avoid damaging your wrist. The direction indicators were like small railway signals. They were operated by a lever on the steering column that moved the signals out from the side of the car. There were no brake lights, so when slowing down the right arm was passed out through the car window and waved up and down. This movement is now sometimes used to hail taxis. Car boots were unusual and many early cars, like the Austin 7, had luggage trunks fastened to the back of the car which could be removed with all their contents as required. I still have the trunk from my grandfather's car. Petrol cost about 5 shillings a gallon (25p in today's currency) while it was £6 a gallon in 2014.

As owning a car enabled my father to commute, we moved to 'Hollow Tree House' in Tardebigge, a rural setting in Worcestershire, about 12 miles outside of Birmingham. There was a real hollow tree in the garden! For the first year or so, I continued at kindergarten in Edgbaston being driven in by my father on his way to work, but travelling home by bus with a parcel label tied around my neck so the driver knew where to put me down. This was in a nearby village called Burcot where my mother collected me. Later I enjoyed the independence of walking the mile home from the bus stop. Fear of child abduction at that time was not common and the last minute 'school run' had not been invented.

Hollow Tree House

This had been built in the early 20th century with two main floors, a two-room attic with sloping roofs and a large underground cellar. The cellar was dark and a bit spooky with wide stone shelving around the edges. A chute came 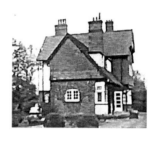 down from ground level through which coke and coal were delivered. Root vegetables and fruit were also stored in the cellar. I learnt how to grow mushrooms in special compost on the cellar shelves. Most family meals were formal with all the family around the table together and once during breakfast there were explosions below the floorboards due to corks being expelled from my father's newly sealed beer bottles. He had bottled the beer while it was still fermenting! In very wet weather, when the water table rose, the cellar would flood to a two-foot depth allowing paddling and sometimes swimming. Recently, when revisiting the house, I was able to reassure the current owners that cellar flooding had been going on for at least 50 years and had never done any harm - clearly the previous owners had chosen not to mention this in the prospectus!

My private space was a bedroom in the attic and large enough for me to lay out my electric 'TRIX' railway, revolutionary at the time because it had 3 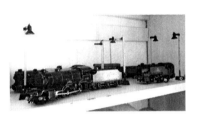 rails allowing 2 engines to run on the track at the same time which, of course, allowed crashes. My first engine is shown here.

I had a mini science laboratory with a microscope and the means of conducting various electrical and chemical experiments. However, in the summer and sometimes the winter, I preferred sleeping outside in an open veranda.

My room was not altogether private however, and when my brother started university he held a party in the house while our parents were away. It was very scary so I 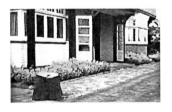 shut myself in my bedroom only to be invaded periodically by couples, who I assumed were exploring. The next day I was upset because my piano, of which I was very fond, had been covered in beer and cigarette ash! My brother had taken a joyride in my father's new car and had an accident, so the police visited the next day, and my parents were not pleased to say the least.

We had a Rayburn multipurpose stove in the kitchen which became the centre of activity during colder months. It burned coke: the by-product of coal that had been heated anaerobically in closed furnaces to release coal gas. This coal gas was stored under pressure in the huge dome shaped gas tanks still seen, usually at the periphery of cities, and used to store oil gas for distribution to homes, schools and factories. My brother suffered from severe asthma and this was before bronchodilator drugs were available. He would regularly inhale menthol from a basin of hot water at the kitchen table beside the Rayburn cooker with a towel over his head listening to Radio Luxembourg. This was one of the very first independent pop music radio stations and was, at that time, illegal. The very first was Radio Caroline transmitted from a small boat in the English Channel.

We now complain about cold weather but then it was just accepted as normal winter weather. With no central heating, ice patterns would appear on the bedroom windows made by 'Jack Frost' and we woke in the mornings with frozen noses. Duvets had not been introduced but well tucked-in sheets and blankets were fine. I enjoyed reading books under the sheets and my favourites were Enid Blyton and Arthur Ransom's adventure stories. I have vivid memories of cycling back from school in snow and ice with freezing blue hands, despite gloves. It seemed to take ages to thaw them out. When it snowed car chains were essential since clearing with snow-ploughs was unusual especially in the country, and salt and sand mixtures were not yet being used on roads. I don't remember this ever meaning I missed school, but it sometimes meant walking or pushing my bike. Pupils were not sent home, as now, if the classrooms were cold. Coats, gloves and extra exercises classes kept us warm.

We had an electric kettle although it was rarely used since the Rayburn supplied hot water. Baths were in rotation or the bathtub was shared. Washing day was Monday and we had a double sink, one for washing and the other for rinsing. There was a mangle to squeeze water out of the clothes before they were hung up outside or on a clothes pulley attached to the kitchen ceiling. I enjoyed turning the mangle handle and when an electrical motor was added I sometimes mangled my fingers, fortunately without permanent injury. Why do we no longer have clothes airing cupboards above our hot water tanks? Probably because many of us now use electricity-hungry tumble driers to take out those last drops of water.

Many houses, including ours, had 'cold stores' or cellars (fridges came later) with thick stonewalls and no windows and often they were partially or completely underground. Fruit, vegetables, butter and cheese were stored here but fresh milk was delivered daily. In our case by the local farmer from a milk churn on the back of his bicycle. He was upset when my father decided that we should use pasteurised milk, to avoid being exposed to bovine tuberculosis, which was only available in reusable milk bottles. This pleased the blue tits because they loved pecking through the foil tops to take out the cream that that risen to the top - no low fat milk in those days.

I remember a telephone being installed and prior to

this it was necessary to go to the post office to make a phone call. If communication was urgent, and the recipient did not have a phone, then the post office would send a telegram that was transmitted using code to the recipient's local post office for delivery. Phone calls, except for

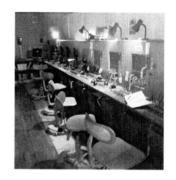

very local ones, had to be connected through the telephone operator (contacted by dialing '0') and direct dialing was not widespread until the end of the 1960s, or in some areas even later. The illustration shows a telephone exchange at the time with the manual 'plug-in' boards to connect the calls. The cost of calls was an issue so my father would give three rings to say he was on his way home - 'woe betide' us if we picked up the phone before it had rung thrice.

One evening my father came home and told us he had a surprise for us, which turned out to be a poliomyelitis vaccine injection. This was hardly exciting, but in retrospect, we were lucky to receive this just as it had become available. My father's dental technician had a severely shortened and deformed leg from poliomyelitis so we knew what the disease could cause. In spite of this, he was a very good swimmer, a skill that he later taught me.

Christmas was a special time but was not commercialised, and became very different when the consumer society kicked-in in the 1960s and 70s. Celebrations started on Christmas Eve when we would put up decorations and prepare for the arrival of Father Christmas by putting our stockings at the end of our beds. In the morning there was normally a silver shilling, a tangerine, some sweets and various small items like balloons, pencils, etc. We received one substantial, normally very useful, present from our parents. One year it was a bicycle and another, my first electric railway set. I remember clearly the sensation of being able to ride round and round the back lawn for the first time and being concerned about how to get off. For many years afterwards I had very pleasant dreams about standing on the lawn, flapping my arms like a bird and then starting to fly for miles between the trees looking down at the earth from above.

The Garden

The garden was about an acre in size and had a huge copper beech tree which was regularly climbed by me and still grows strong 60 years later. There was a large bamboo shrubbery that allowed passages and dens to be created. Arthur Ransom enthusiasts will realise why I enjoyed his books such as 'Swallows and Amazons' so much. My father, who had become proficient before and during the War in growing vegetables, (he also loved roses and wallflowers) continued these skills, eventually developing a very productive vegetable area. A highlight was picking and eating crops such as peas and raspberries direct from the plants. I had my own garden patch and found carrots, peas, onions, broad beans and new potatoes were the easiest to grow. The soil was very heavy due to its clay content, but mixed with garden and animal compost as well as lime, it became highly fertile.

My adventurousness led me once to picking damsons from the top of a tree where they got most sun, and in the process fell backwards off a tall ladder. I woke up in the house 5 or 10 minutes later with my anxious mother looking over me. 'Knocking yourself out' was not uncommon and did not normally then result in spending a night in hospital under observation, as is the case now. Maybe I was lucky, but my medically trained father kept a close eye on me.

Bee Keeping

We lived next to a large apple orchard so my mother tried bee keeping, but gave it up when she reacted badly to stings. I later followed her example and have now kept bees for more than 30 years with plenty of stings but nothing too serious. I suspect my mother was not truly anaphylactic but had nasty local reactions to the venom. Most beekeepers find this a problem at the beginning of a season but after a few stings the reaction tends to subside.

Chickens

There was space for me to keep chickens and at one stage I sold the eggs for pocket money. I did this either at the doorstep to passers-by or at a small stall in the nearby farmers market. I think most of my customers bought the eggs to encourage me although on one occasion I won second prize for '6 brown eggs' at our local church and village fete! Humanely dispatching hens that were ill, very old or unproductive by breaking their neck in an instant was an essential skill. Even now I get summoned by friends to help when they require this service for their, usually very small, domestic flocks. Experiments with keeping geese failed because they tended to drown themselves in any easily available water tubs and were also very messy because they predominantly eat grass that only gets partially digested. I learnt not to like foxes, to put it mildly, after I once left the henhouse door unbolted at night only to find my whole flock of 60 hens decimated in the morning. As well as taking eggs to the local market, I sold apples, brambles, blackberries and fruit picked from our neighbour's farm's hedgerows.

Rabbits

I kept and bred angora rabbits as pets and for their fur which was sold on for making woollen garments. Keeping them mostly in cages meant regular feeding and cleaning was necessary. Later I used to have occasional nightmares that I had forgotten to feed them, but they always seemed, in my dreams, to have survived this ordeal. By contrast, wild rabbits were a big problem both for farmers and gardeners. My father had 'dug for victory' very effectively during the War but this was in a city where there were neither foxes nor rabbits. In the country, large colonies would destroy fields of wheat and vegetables by progressively eating their way into fields from their burrows in bordering hedges or woodland. However, rabbits were an important source of meat and at harvest time, when the corn was being cut in circles from the hedges inwards, rabbits were forced further and further towards the remaining central patch of corn. They would then rush out in all directions to a hail of pellets from shotguns. I was once hit by stray pellets when eating a sandwich at the edge of the field but fortunately sustained no injuries!

In the garden we tied wire netting to secure the edge, but it never seemed to work. Snares were popular but cruel. Nothing effectively controlled rabbit populations until the government released the viral infection, myxomatosis, which quickly decimated the whole country's rabbit population. Some of these infected rabbits survive and develop immunity so the infection is still around. Then the numbers increase every 5-10 years sufficiently for a new non-immune population to build up so the disease starts to spread again. My angora rabbits were vaccinated.

Guinea Pigs, Stick Insects, Budgerigars, Birds Eggs and Butterflies

I also kept guinea pigs - not for food! Unlike rabbits, whose young are born blind and hairless, guinea pig young are fully formed at birth and look and behave immediately just like miniature adults. They breed incessantly with at least 6 or 8 in each litter so finding them new homes could be a problem.

My Aunt Christine introduced me to stick insects

and budgerigars. She was one of the very first PhD biology teachers in Scotland and her classroom was full of plants and insects of varying types as well as tadpoles, fish and budgerigars; she used to teach her pupils about genetics. She was a highly respected teacher and was passionate about her subject. Sadly, when her school became a comprehensive, she took early retirement as she found it too difficult to adjust to teaching teenagers, many of whom had little background or interest in her subject. With her help, I decided to build a budgie-shed myself attached to an aviary and had some breeding success. Like rabbits, baby budgies are very skinny, blind and naked when born. I never really liked keeping animals or birds in cages so I experimented with letting the budgies loose during the days to explore nearby trees and shrubs. I think they ended up being a good source of protein for local cats and hawks.

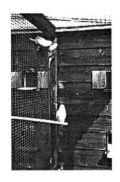

In those days there were no laws against collecting wild bird's eggs so I had quite a collection built up over several years. Watching where birds flew into hedges helped identify their nests and egg collecting was strictly a case of 'only one' from any one nest and no duplicates. These days, most children will only see the beautiful variations in wild birds eggs at museums. Irresponsible egg collecting is clearly to be discouraged, but it is surely the destruction of hedges that has taken more of a toll on bird populations than egg collecting. I also had quite an extensive collection of preserved butterflies which were much more common, as they were not killed by all the insecticides used on our farms and in our gardens today.

Steam Train Spotting

Many think of Worcestershire as a rural county with rolling countryside, cattle, cereal and fruit farms. However, Hollow Tree House was within easy walking distance of the steepest 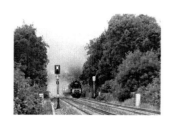 mainline railway in England called the Lickey Incline and also the Tardebigge Canal, with a tunnel over 500 yards long and cut through solid rock.

Much time however, was spent train spotting with a friend, Keith Rockevans, watching the steam engines struggle up or race down the Lickey Incline. There was nothing comparable to watching these huge and complicated steam monsters doing their work with all the moving engine parts on display. It is difficult to describe the excitement of a train approaching up the incline with its noise, smoke and steam,

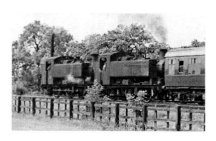 followed by watching it pass by within yards while waving to the driver and guard! You could see their smoke and steam from a long distance away and put

your ear onto the lines to hear the rails rattling as they approached. There was the well-known 'clickety-click' sound, now usually only heard on films, when the wheels in groups of four or six crossed over short gaps between the rails. This gap was intentional to allow the rails to expand on hot days without buckling the tracks. Later on rails were lengthened, I think due to using steel treated to minimize expansion, which was the demise of this typical steam train sound. Some tracks in Scotland still 'clickety-click' such as the line between Inverness and Kyle of Lochalsh and the sound carries for miles across water when the line goes along the Moray Firth.

There were many different types and sizes of steam engines and they all had unique numbers and many had names which allowed us to keep records of those we had seen. It is hard to describe the 'personalities' steam engines had to those born after the 1950s, but it has been said they are machines with human attributes. That is, they need food (coal) and water, whistle to you, make various chugging and rattling noises, often skid on the track when they start and the cranks and pistons seem like arms and legs. Diesel engines have none of this romance and the engine and moving parts are hidden from sight. There were even special carriages used for sorting Royal Mail letters and parcels, and special apparatus on the side of mail carriages which picked up and delivered sacks of letters and parcels while the train was on the move. We got to know some of the engines very well since they were regulars on the line.

The banker engines helped push the trains up the

incline from behind when the
engines at the front could not
cope. One especially powerful
banker was called 'Big Bertha'
(illustrated). Sometimes two
small bankers for one train were
necessary. In 1840 a banker

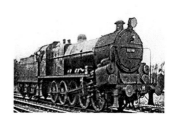

engine's boiler exploded with the effort, resulting in the loss
of the lives of the driver and fireman. They are buried in
Bromsgrove Church graveyard. After trains had passed us
by and reached the top of the incline the bankers returned
backwards down the incline to help push up the next train.
Occasionally the drivers would stop and we were allowed
to ride on the footplate of the engine and blow the whistle.
I doubt if this would be approved of now without formal
permission and many health and safety checks!

Steam engines used the best quality coal and quite
a lot fell off their coal bunkers into the fields on the sides
of the track where we would collect it and make campfires.
Another game was crushing penny coins into flat discs by
putting them on the line before a train was due to pass.
Much of this thrill of the steam engine will be recognised by
enthusiasts of the book and films of 'The Railway Children'
or similar novels.

When we witnessed the first diesel engine, with
its rather boring appearance, using the incline we did not
realise at the time this was going to be the demise of the
steam engines. Nor did we realise that most trains pulled
by diesels did not require bankers except for those with

numerous heavy goods trucks. Now the few that are left mostly run on separate tracks as tourist attractions. It had been decided by the government of the time that cars and lorry transport were to be encouraged at the expense of the railways. We got to know the 'bankers' and their drivers and firemen well.

Fishing

I spent much time canal-fishing using floats and maggots which is very different from the fly-fishing common in Scotland. Small, but edible, bream and the occasional aggressive pike were the most common catches. Sitting quietly on a stool, waiting for a bite, was an introduction to meditation but also allowed observation of birds, water voles and other wildlife. The canals were not at this time being used extensively for barge holidays, which eventually made successful float fishing on them difficult. Later, as an infectious diseases doctor, I became involved in recognising that these voles and water rats could spread a potentially lethal infection called hantaan fever, as well as the better known leptospirosis or Weil's disease.

Entertainment in the Home

There was no mass media, except for radio and newspapers, and reading was important. As explained earlier, often reading was under the bedclothes by torchlight due to strict 'go to sleep' times. Home-made crystal radio sets were great fun, very small, needed no batteries and easily picked up the main BBC and some continental radio stations.

During this continuation of post-war austerity, manufactured toys were a luxury and were usually made of wood or cardboard. More often we played with home-made toys and used our imagination making dens, pretend cars and boats out of old boxes or furniture. I remember being very upset when I damaged the top of a small table in my Uncle Eric's house. I had it upside down and was pushing my sister in it around the carpet, pretending to be a train driver. Eric was immediately forgiving.

In the 1950s model railways were popular. Initially wooden ones with 'chains with chucks' on rails, then ones driven by clockwork motors wound-up with a key like the ones we still use for wind-up clocks. Then came electric model railways including Hornby, which has stood the test of time. It was predictable that my interest in train spotting, as described previously, led me to have my own model railway 'TRIX' set. The special thing about the 'TRIX' system was that 2 trains could be run independently because the track had a central negative rail with the side rails feeding electricity to the 2 separate engines. There was an obvious risk of accidents so driving skills were important and the tracks had to be designed carefully with passing places as well as side tracks for parking. Stations, buildings and tunnels were made up from cardboard printed sheets and glued together. The other essential skill was some knowledge of electrical wiring and the use of transformers. I also had a small steam engine where the water was heated by a methylated spirit burner.

While television was invented in the 1930s, it only became widespread in homes in the 1950s and like many others we got a 'tele' to watch the coronation of Queen Elizabeth ll in 1953 with our neighbours. This was a very big event with village street parties, numerous souvenirs, extra school holidays and I still have my commemorative silver coin. To have more than one television set was virtually unheard of, maybe partly because the set was the size of a small chest of drawers and the screen the size of a dinner plate. There was only one channel initially and no commercial advertising. ITV began broadcasting in 1955 and later BBC 2 in 1964. The inside of the set was full of exciting things called 'valves' which were hot and glowed. Transmission was twice a day, with an hour of children's programmes after school such as 'Muffin the Mule', 'The Flower Pot Men' and later 'Blue Peter'. After 7pm, evening news and other programmes for adults were shown ending around 10.30pm. Frequently the picture was interrupted and a screen would come up saying, 'Sorry for the inconvenience, normal transmission will resume as soon as possible' - often seemingly during the most exciting part of a film! Morning television only began in the late 1960s and was very controversial because it was thought it might make people late for school or work.

Through the 20th and 21st centuries relaxation and play activities for children have altered dramatically. Perhaps the most obvious change is the availability of plastic toys and games. I became very aware of this change recently when a friend and I opened a recycling charity shop for second hand children's clothes, toys and books, most of which would have otherwise gone to landfill sites or be stored under beds or in lofts. This made me wonder about the implications of the ever-popular model cars and what they do to children's ways of thinking about environmental issues as they all seem to be fantasy models, racing cars or 'gas guzzlers'. Many modern board games appear very complicated, and are often sold in large boxes with little inside. They seem to be often given as presents by well-intentioned parents and relatives thinking they might have educational value, but are actually used very little.

Outside The Home

This included going to the 'pictures' before the days of television. Since the advent of television, many of these cinemas have been demolished or converted into bingo halls. Attending the 'pictures' was an exciting adventure; ticket queues, rows of comfortable seats, cigarette smoke and ushers with ice cream baskets around their necks. The 'shorts' featured news stories, largely concerning the royalty and the military and the sound level did not require ear plugs, as it seems to nowadays.

In the 1960s coffee bars became popular usually with a jukebox into which we put 6 pence (240 to the pound) or a shilling to play our favourite pop tunes. The jive arrived in Britain during the War, learnt from the many African-American servicemen based here, and was followed by rock and roll. I have never fully understood why these very lively, structured and enjoyable dance forms, largely vanished into do-what-you-like dances which have become the norm in modern-day nightclubs. Maybe this has something to do with heavy alcohol drinking now being synonymous with 'a good night out' and after a few pints it is no longer possible to dance using any sort of structured technique! Later in my teenage years, I came to enjoy jazz and joined a club where dancing was probably halfway between jive and modern disco style. Once, when I was about 10 years old, I was sent to traditional ballroom dancing classes that were fun but you had to hold onto girls, which was scary! I stopped going when the girl I had confidence dancing with decided she wanted a change of partner. Then there was Elvis, Teddy Boys, winkle pickers and The Beatles. In Scotland, of course, we have our own traditional ceilidh dancing which has stood the test of time and even seems to be becoming popular in England.

Outdoor children's activities have changed and not just because of the advent of computers, but through fear of allowing children do what might be called 'risky' activities. This seems to have resulted from a widespread concern about letting children do things unsupervised and has extended to a fear of letting children walk or cycle to school following wide media coverage of abductions and accidents. I have no idea whether these risks have increased or whether they are just more widely reported. Health and safety regulations aim to encourage parents and others to take common sense precautions but they often seem to be interpreted as forbidding many of the activities from which children can learn about taking sensible degrees of risk. So much learning, communicating and entertainment now is in front of a television or computer screen rather than from risk-taking itself.

Memorable Family Holidays Around This Time

Package holidays had not been invented except for Butlin's seaside camps and Thomas Cook's overseas trips mostly by train or bus, so our holidays in early childhood were visiting relatives in Scotland. An exception for us was a bus trip to Oberammergau in Bavaria to see the famous outdoor 'Passion Play' depicting the last days in the life of Jesus. The play, the hotel and the mountains were exciting but the long bus trip very tedious. My father asked the bus driver whether there was a toilet and was told, "No. Just the back window"! This left a lot to the imagination.

Seaside Trips to Ayr

Because it was my parent's birthplace, most family holidays were in Scotland and we often stayed with my mother's parents who lived in a small bungalow near the beach in Ayr. These trips involved getting up at around 5am and driving up the West Coast of England along the A6. This was before there were any motorways and the route went through the centre of towns like Wolverhampton, Lancaster, Penrith and Carlisle. It usually took us about 10 hours. Having 100% 'Scottish blood', as we called it, we would cheer when we saw the 'Welcome to Scotland' signs and 'boo' on the way back when we saw the 'Welcome to England' signs! Not because of any nationalist tendencies, just because it felt like 'going home'. Interestingly, for these journeys we had to wear smart trousers, a shirt, tie and jacket. What are now called 'T' shirts and jeans did not become popular until the 1960s. Trips down to the beach and the nearby ice cream shop on the shore run by Mr Seekie were highlights. The donkey rides have now been replaced by racehorses and pleasure riders galloping along the beach. I hardly remember it ever raining which is thought to be because Ayr is in a 'rain shadow' from the mountains on the Isle of Arran, which is about 5 miles offshore.

In those days town councils owned most Scottish golf courses and rounds were very cheap so we learnt some of the skills; 'slow back swing and keep your head down until you have hit the ball'. Some say golf was invented in Scotland but others say Holland, which had close trading links with the east of Scotland including the famous golf centre of St Andrews.

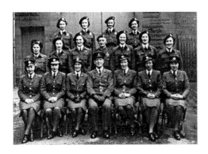

My grandfather was awarded the 'Member of the British Empire' medal for services during World War II as head of the local aircraft observer corps. He used to take me into town on a Saturday morning and disapproved of the traffic in the main street because he considered pedestrians should have priority. He would raise his walking stick and set off across the road expecting the traffic to stop! There was a shop down a side street where he bought oatmeal for our porridge - it had to be very finely ground and then soaked overnight before cooking. His favorite sport was bowls. I came to realise, without any understanding of the reasons, that he was quite strongly anti-royalist and probably would have been an enthusiastic member of the Scottish National Party if it had existed at the time. My grandmother was much less active and walked with a limp for as long as I knew her. She had been one the first people to have a hip replacement for arthritis and it was not wholly successful. She understandably refused to go for any further surgery. Perhaps because of my postwar infancy when my mother was on her own while my father was in India and my rather stressful school experiences, I have always tended towards being overanxious. Even as a teenager my grandmother used to say I was an 'accident looking for somewhere to happen!'

I was very fond of my grandparents, who were very kind to us, but remember being quite shocked, at my grand-fathers reaction, when it was reported that a senior politician in London had become embroiled in a spy scandal involving a prostitute and he committed suicide. My grandfather said that he thought this was the best outcome (unless I misunderstood him). Everything went quiet when I responded that I thought this was an awful thing to say, after which I was I reprimanded by my father who said that there is a time and a place for expressing these sort of views. Today this sort of openness of expression by a 16 year old may well be encouraged.

In 1914 a new Sunday newspaper, the Sunday Post, was launched with the aim of keeping the public informed about the First World War and to publish lighthearted, morale-boosting articles. The paper is still going strong and has become something of a Scottish institution. Because it was not available in England, every week my grandfather would wrap up his copy after he had read it and post it to my mother. There was, and still is, a children's section with cartoon stories depicting life in Scotland called 'Oor Wullie' and 'The Broons'. I was a big fan and still am.

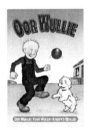 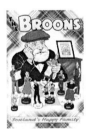

Solway Adventures

Later, during teenage years, our holidays were still in Scotland but centered on Ashlands, a small guesthouse in Rockcliffe on the Solway coast. I still have film footage that my father took with his very early film camera. This included line fishing for flounders which involved digging up lugworms from the mud at low tide and hanging them

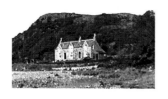 from hooks onto a line hung between two stakes firmly stuck in the mud. We would get up very early and follow the tide going out to see if we had caught anything before the gulls could come down to steal the catch. Catching conger eels from cracks and crevices in rocks, normally never exposed, was only possible at very low tides. Collecting brambles with our landlady's daughter, Annabel, and boiling them up on a little stove in the back shed before filtering the mixture to make bramble 'wine' was a highlight! Morning papers and post were brought to the village on a local bus and thrown by the driver from his seat to the door of the local post offices for delivery.

Expeditions incorporated into stays at Rockcliffe included going to the Edinburgh Military Tattoo and a weeks driving up the West Coast of Scotland with a caravan that once disconnected itself from the car before rolling backwards into a ditch on a single-track road. In the Highlands the majority of the roads were then single track and the numerous ferries across river estuaries are now mostly replaced by bridges including one 'over the sea' to Skye. Much of this was recorded on my father's film and the very special historical 'snap' shown is of the large Ullapool fishing fleet, now replaced by modern diesel powered boats, in the harbour with their very distinctive black square sails.

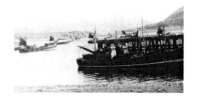

WORK ON THE FARM
INTEGRATED WITH NATURE

Much of my spare time during teenage years was spent helping and working on our neighbour's farm. This was a very special time for me, partly the experience of 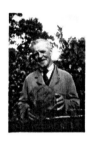 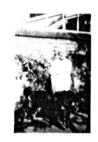 working on the land and with animals, but also because of the very close relationship I developed with Ed Hall and his parents. I was especially close to Nancy, his mother, who was always known to me as 'Mrs Hall'. They had an old dog called 'Merry' who was an excellent rat catcher but at other times was as friendly and calm as it is possible to imagine. Today we might call their farm 'traditional' or 'organic'. These words were not widely used in the 1950s as the application of oil based and chemical fertilizers on farms, as well as monoculture, were not normal practice. Our tasks included husbandry for a wide variety of animals and crops, working with nature, rather than trying to control it.

At the time I naively never considered that there could be any other approaches to farm management than a love of and respect for nature. Soil, plants, animals, microorganisms and the weather; all natures components working together. It was just accepted that all these elements work in balance with some winners and some losers, in what we now understand as an ecosystem. Today most farming is a business aiming to maximise output and increase profits. It is dependent upon finite chemical resources, and is at the cost of long-term soil fertility.

We had about five milking cows. Friesians, Herefords and Shorthorns which were all milked by hand. We made our own butter. The cattle were kept out on grass except if there was deep snow when they were brought under cover. Since continual milk production depends upon a cow regularly having a new calf, about 3 months after calving when the cow becomes receptive, a chosen bull was brought to the farm. This has now been largely replaced by artificial insemina- 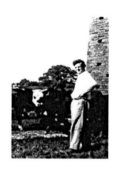 tion. I regularly helped with milking and routine care to a point where I was sometimes proudly left on my own in charge for a weekend. I have always found opening jars with tight lids easy, which I put down to strong fingers from regular milking!

It wasn't going to be long before farming subsidies and a government funded milk marketing board were created to increase production and give a guaranteed price to farmers for certain products such as milk and wheat. This resulted in a move from smaller multipurpose farms, supplying local needs, to intensive farming that focused on just one or two crops. In Scotland these were wheat, oats and barley. More recently rape has become popular as have specific breeds of cattle, pigs, sheep or chickens (usually in battery cages).

There was a decline in the traditional cattle breeds that had been adjusted to the local pasture and climate conditions. Many established breeds were replaced in these new-style farms by very high yield genetically designed ones such as the Holstein, and understandably many farmers made this switch to benefit from the fixed subsidised income. However, there was a price to pay as the new breeds developed arthritic and sterility problems, and eventually there was gross overproduction of milk and milk products throughout Europe. These 'butter mountains' led to the demise of the guaranteed price. Locally adjusted breeds are now becoming more popular again and there is a move, albeit limited, towards the older systems of sustainable farm management.

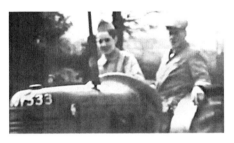

This was around the time when horses were being replaced by tractors for the tasks of ploughing, harrowing, rolling, scything, harvesting, grass cutting and transporting items around the farm. I drove a small John Brown or Ferguson tractor and carried out all these tasks. Pictured opposite is one of my straight furrows! My tractor had none of the comforts of air-conditioned, enclosed cabins complete with wi-fi, heating and kettles they have today.

We just got wet, cold (or hot) and wind-swept which I can't help feeling was somehow healthier.

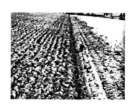

Ploughing took longer because we only used 2 or 3 plough-shares instead of the 6 to 10 used now by very large tractors that incidentally greatly compress the ground, making ploughing even more necessary! All the fields were small and surrounded by hedges full of wildlife (looking for birds' nests and rabbit, fox or badger burrows was a favourite pastime). Most hedges have since been uprooted, making fields larger. The hedges have been replaced by wire and netting boundaries to allow faster and easier access for larger, less manoeuvrable machinery.

We kept pigs, chickens and pigeons. Wheat, potatoes and grass were the main soil crops and hedgerows included a variety of fruit trees. Hedges needed regular maintenance, cutting and 'layering'; binding branches together to make a stock proof barrier. Hedges that remain are usually now roughly cut back by machine, which inevitably leaves holes near the foot of the hedge for stock to escape through, and so additional wire netting is needed.

In addition to the physical work and the learning of many farming skills, much of my enjoyment came from feeling my work was appreciated. I was also aware that teaching gave Ed much pleasure which was in contrast to my experience with many of my school teachers!

I have mentioned previously how the proximity to the War still affected everyone. Ed could describe vividly the dogfights over his land that he had witnessed during the Battle of Britain. His mother would describe with passion how Churchill's speeches were listened to regularly, and were a major factor in maintaining morale.

Mrs Hall showed me how to make a good cup of tea: the water had to continue to boil after the tea leaves and a spoon of sugar were added. Tea bags had not been invented and, when they were, they seemed very wasteful when they were used to make just one small cup of not very tasty tea! She had her special chair, in the small living room, next to the fire which was the only source of heat in the house and would always stand to wave goodbye at the gate. Her favourite flowers were lily of the valley and there was a specially cared for cluster outside the farmhouse backdoor. Once, at Christmas, she introduced me to her home-made parsnip wine. This was my first experience of alcohol and I can still recollect that wobbly feeling when walking home and trying to cross the road safely.

Mr Hall senior, died from bowel cancer not long after the picture was taken of us on a tractor. As described later, Mrs Hall died after a stroke while I was at university, and Ed lived till he was in his eighties. Interestingly, there was never any question of any of the family spending their last days in hospital and they were all cared for at home in contrast from usual terminal care practice now in the UK. This was more like the practice in India, which I describe later, when dying patients were usually taken home when in extremis by their relatives even if this involved train journeys.

All Change

Unsurprisingly, I wished for a career in agriculture and had a place in agricultural college. However, after being accepted into college and working as an apprentice on a diary farm that only dealt in milk and beef production, I found myself becoming disillusioned. I realised that business

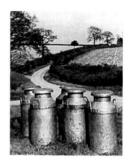

farming, focusing first on profit, did not appeal to me. I was paid £3 a week for starting at 5am and finishing around 7pm with a bonus of £3 at Christmas. It had been much more fun working on the Hall's farm for no pay but much appreciation. I would have preferred to do my apprenticeship with the Halls but their farm was not recognised as suitably modern by the college. However, the experience was useful and I learnt the skills of milking by machine, cleaning out milking parlors and helping cows to deliver their calves. Initially Mr Hall delivered milk to local households from a container carried around on the back of his bicycle. Then came milk churns transferring milk to the 'milk' factories firstly by horse and cart and then lorries where it was sterilised and bottled. I was even introduced to Woodbine cigarettes by one of the farm hands who was a German soldier during the War. He had stayed on in England after he had been released from prisoner-of-war camp.

These developing doubts with regards to a career in modern farming were in my mind when I had a car accident involving a double somersault in one of the cattle farm's poorly maintained trucks. I landed upside down at the foot of a bank on the side of a narrow road. This was before the days of MOTs and seat belts. I was told my immediate, somewhat dazed, concern was to sweep the broken glass off the road so that other cars would not be damaged. My parents were away that weekend and it was Mrs Hall that looked after me.

The truck was a write-off, and the visit to hospital for stitches somehow prompted me to consider switching to medicine. My father was not keen and he seemed to doubt my intellectual abilities, but my Uncle Eric quietly took me aside and suggested that perhaps this was meant for me, giving me the necessary courage to make the switch. I had no problem being accepted into medical school since I had the correct 'A' level exams results and at the interview they seemed fascinated with my having left school early, gone to a higher education college and my love of the countryside more so than my commitment to a medical career!

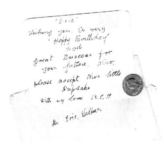

When I eventually left home to go to medical school, Mrs Hall gave me a card and golden sovereign with a pencil 'dot' in the middle of the envelope saying that the farm would be 'a lonely spot'. I treasure this still.

She died suddenly about 3 years later from a stroke shortly before Ed was planning to marry. When Ed rang me, without thinking about the time or distance (about 12 miles), I cycled immediately to the farm in the dark from my University Hall of Residence in Birmingham. More, I believe, to control my emotions than to especially share immediate condolences with Ed, although obviously this played a part.

The Farming 'Revolution'

I have already described the rather dramatic changes to farming practice which occurred during the 1950s by the introduction of government farm subsidies to encourage specialisation and maximum production. This meant that government and retail outlets exerted more control over what farmers produced and the methods they used. Quantity and profit began to take priority over producing varieties of healthy food, much of which was sold at local markets for local consumption. This led to the current practice of wasting large quantities of otherwise excellent produce because it does not have a colour and shape that supermarkets think are necessary to please customers. I challenge someone to find 'carrots in love' on a supermarket shelf.

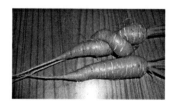

It has also led to a lot of less popular but excellent foods having to be imported from abroad. This practice however, can encourage producers in poorer countries to concentrate on exports rather than growing essential supplies for their local villages. It also adds to environmental pollution and climate change with all the air and sea transport required.

Today's continual 'monoculture' (repeatedly growing the same crops on the same land) results in the quality of soil deteriorating and requires repeated use of chemicals to maintain fertility and replace vital minerals. The structure of the soil also changes, losing its crumbly nature full of humus, microorganisms and worms. We only need to dig up a sample of soil managed in the modern way and compare it with soil from a small field which is surrounded by hedges and trees (allowing leaves and organic debris, fungi, insect and animal droppings to abound) to appreciate the difference.

The move from horses to machinery has meant the demise of the local village blacksmith. Who, along with caring for horses hoofs and shoes, was highly skilled in making harnesses and repairing agricultural equipment such as carts, ploughs, harrows, rollers, pitchforks, spades and shovels. Agricultural engineers now look after farm machinery and horses feet are looked after at home by specialised farriers with bottle gas powered mini-furnaces carried around in small vans. They serve much larger geographical areas since there is no need to take the horse to the blacksmith. Many horse owners think the personalised expert craftsmanship skills have been lost in a similar way to our loss of the local family doctor.

Harvesting corn has ceased to be a community event. Farmers worked together in teams often going straight from one farm to another. Sheaves of corn were cut and bound by hand, or using a tractor and simple mechanical scythe driven by its wheels rotating on the ground. They were then stacked or 'stooked' in clusters of six sheaves to dry. The gain was then separated from the straw by mechanical or hand thrashing. During my 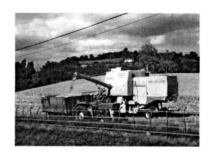 latter days on the Hall's farm, the combine harvester replaced this largely manual process. When combine harvesters are used, the grain has to be dry before harvesting or else it needs to be dried in heated driers involving extra expense. This is another example of how machinery designed for mass-production changed farming methods and increases our dependency on fossil fuel energy. 'Mass-production' is a term used to mean saving time, reducing the number of workers required and increasing profit. However, I doubt if this substantially increases the amount of grain and straw produced long-term. Fertility of the soil together with the weather (which is outside our control) are much more important for long-term sustainability. Monoculture quickly leads to deserted land (deserts) when the soil quality has deteriorated, water has run out and man moves on.

Passionate Interests Don't Die!

Working on Ed's farm, caring for livestock, ploughing, harrowing, seed planting and harvesting well into the night until it was too dark to continue, are still experiences I recollect when needing to relax and let my mind escape from the pressures of today's hectic and often unavoidably chaotic but modern ways of living.

Since these early days, my connection with farming and horticulture has continued in various ways. I have grown vegetables in any local available ground. As a junior doctor, when living in rural India, and when I was doing my general practice training in Worcestershire; I cultivated vegetables. In Scotland, we rented a tumbledown farmhouse (much to the disapproval of the in-laws but approval of the children) and now live in another very old farmhouse attached to a converted byre (cowshed). We have 3 acres of land for vegetable and fruit production, and grazing for animals as needed. A large field pond encourages other wildlife such as ducks, frogs, fish, toads, herons, voles and the occasional osprey.

EDUCATION IN THE 1950S - MIXED EXPERIENCES

In the 1940s and 1950s schooling had 3 stages - kindergarten from 4-5 years, primary school from 8 years and senior school from the age of 12. The school leaving age was from 15 years.

Kindergarten

Many schools in Birmingham had been destroyed by bombing, or taken over for military purposes during the war and my kindergarten was held in an adapted residential house. The 'basics' of reading, writing and arithmetic predominated, augmented by an introduction to an additional wide range of subjects. I revelled in nature study and one summer won the class prize for the largest collection of pressed wild flowers. We regularly took our pets such as dogs, rabbits and guinea pigs into school. A highlight was a large metal climbing frame on the lawn in the back garden, which we used in break times.

Mrs MacGeough ran the kindergarten in a friendly family atmosphere in complete contrast to my later school experiences. We all looked forward to our third of a pint of milk at break times. I remember fainting once when standing up to read when I had a fever, and I was well looked after. The girls' classrooms were in a neighbouring house and I remember being very concerned about my younger sister when she had just started school and I had to be taken across to see that she was all right and not crying!

There was a wall chart for overall achievements, and one year I came top and went through a scary award ceremony where all the children dressed up as Knights of the Round Table. I was 'knighted' with a grey wooden sword, which I was given to keep, but sadly it disappeared later after I had left home when my parents were having a clear out. I don't think they realised its significance to me.

Primary School

Starting real school was a shock. I cannot say I ever really settled into the strict and authoritarian regimes that were the norm, especially in private fee-paying 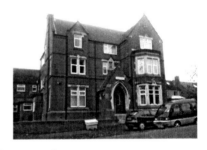 schools during this post-War period.

Both junior and senior schools were designed for boarders, while day-boys like me were in the minority and that made us different. The contrast with kindergarten could not have been more extreme. It was, with few exceptions, a case of everything focused on repeating what we were taught without question, and on following rules and regulations. Classes involved receiving instructions and if you did not get good marks in the regular tests, this led to punishments such as 'lines', detention or beatings. I often feigned sore throats to stay off school, and this resulted in me having my tonsils removed! In general, my experiences of school were rather negative.

These were the days of fountain pens and inkwells. Ballpoint pens were not widely available and they were unreliable, leaked and were very expensive. I still have a nostalgic yearning to return to using a fountain pen which was filled up with 'Quink' ink from inkwells which were incorporated into our desks.

Our mathematics teacher was renowned for shouting, and throwing chalk and board dusters around the room at boys he thought were inattentive. English classes focused on spelling and grammar, and history was a case of reading course books in turn during class with no explanation or discussion. We were required to learn a chapter as homework, were tested on it the following day, and earned detention if we scored less that 50%. I found learning Latin very stressful because it all seemed so strange. Once, I was so upset by it, I was found crying on my own by the headmaster. He gave me some sympathy but then told the teacher involved, which made my fear of Latin even worse.

There was much uncontrolled bullying ranging from picking on certain boys (usually the shy ones), to 'beating up' and physical abuse of a nature that I find difficult to describe in writing. I suspect regular punishments and beatings of pupils by staff for misdemeanors encouraged this sort of behaviour. Going to the toilet was a nightmare since the toilets were outdoor, not private and had no locks. The bullies seemed to congregate there. There was a patch of ground where boys made tracks, bridges and tunnels to play on with their miniature Dinky model cars. There was a very distinct hierarchy defining who could participate. This was also a focus for other problems and once, a boy got hold of an air gun that he fired at others to maintain the bullies' rule of order. Someone was shot between the eyes and could have been blinded. Fortunately, the teachers found out because the victim's forehead was bleeding. I cycled to school from the age of 10 but enjoyed going home best!

It was not bullying as such, but I found it very disturbing one day when a death sentence was reported in the news and about to be carried out (this was still legal in the UK in the 1950s). Some of the boys got together in the school playground to count down to the dedicated time, 12 noon, so they could cheer at the final moment. I suppose in days gone the spectacle of public executions attracted crowds, motivated by a variety of reasons, but it was this apparent enjoyment involving just young children which I found frightening.

There were exceptions to this overall harsh situation. I felt I could relax during optional carpentry lessons, choir and Scouting, after school classes had finished. I enjoyed the practical nature of carpentry classes, taught by a local carpenter. For singing, boys were auditioned and separated into choir A or choir B: school singers and 'growlers'. I had a good sense of tone and pitch so joined choir A. This provided opportunities for out-of-school events, including adding treble voices to the senior school choir. Sometimes choir allowed us to miss other classes, and I sang the first verses of 'Once in Royal David's City' and 'In the Bleak Midwinter' as a solo from the pulpit in the town church. The vicar was very complimentary!

Out of school, I joined the local town church bell ringers with a friend. This required skill and some strength to balance the bells at the top of their rotation, just sufficiently long to change the order of the peal.

Senior School

The atmosphere in the senior school was similar. Absolute obedience to staff was the rule and the reward for asking 'why' was usually punishment. A difference from primary school was that when older boys were made prefects, they took on a similar role in maintaining discipline to staff, presumably to try to teach them leadership skills. 'Fagging', where prefects were allocated a junior boy to carry out tasks for them like shoe cleaning, conveying messages, fetching snacks from the school tuck-shop and running various other errands, was a common practice. A problem was that many of the prefects did not follow the rules themselves and 'discipline' turned into another form of bullying. Prefects were allowed to beat younger boys whenever they wished.

Day-boys were all members of the same house and had to be at the school by 8.30am for a chapel service. We left for home at around 6.30pm after an hour's 'lock-up' to do our homework. I regularly escaped this for choir practice, and in any case, I was allowed away early to catch the last bus home. There were 4 wooden prefabricated lock-up rooms in the grounds into which boys were allocated by year of study. Just before I left school at the age of 15, I was put in charge of Room 3. My main activity in Room 3 was playing chess and we also had a quarter size billiard table upon which I excelled for some reason. I feel it is a shame that billiards as a spectacle has been largely replaced by snooker which, unlike billiards, involves scoring only by potting balls or because of errors by your opponent. Many are now unaware of the skills of 'cannons' and 'in-offs' which also gain points in billiards. In snooker, it is avoiding 'in-offs' that is important, but the skill in estimating striking angles and the resulting direction of travel of the balls is the same.

For two hours after lunch we had sports which included compulsory cricket, rugby, cross-country running and athletics, with tennis and boxing being optional. I enjoyed cricket and was quite good at batting, but the teacher umpire treated it a bit like a mathematics class so we were vociferously told-off if we missed a catch or got run-out. Tennis was fun when playing with friends and it often let you off cross-country running or team sports which seemed to me to be bullying on a playing field. However, my regular cycling to school and farm work kept me fit, so I was able to score tries in rugby by outrunning the opposition. I also did well in long-distance running. I was made to box on one occasion, but could not hit the other person. I ended up with a bleeding nose and a black eye so the teacher decided boxing was not my scene!

This was only 10 years after World War II and we all had to join the Combined Cadet Force (CCF) that was a junior form of army recruitment, until the school decided that Scouts could be exempt. This involved army discipline, inspections, marching, parades, day and night mock exercises including the use of rifles with blank ammunition. We were given our own khaki uniforms and were responsible for the cleaning of our belts, gaiters and badges. Rifle practice with live ammunition was carried out in a special shooting range and, to my surprise, I was awarded a first class shooting badge for accuracy! I quite enjoyed the CCF, I think because everyone was treated the same and we were given clear boundaries for what we could, or could not, do. Major Masseter, who was in charge, often congratulated us when we performed well. Obligatory national service from the age of 18 years was discontinued in 1960, so I missed this by one year, although I think in retrospect medical students were exempt.

Sex education was non-existent and there were many misconceptions over what sex was all about. Sexual activity in all forms was clearly considered 'wrong'. Baden-Powell, in his first edition of 'Scouting for Boys', wrote that self-abuse must be avoided (meaning masturbation), although this paragraph was removed in later editions. I was aware of boys with a homosexual orientation and liaisons seemed to usually take place in toilets. Whether this gay orientation continued into adult life I do not know. Once, a boarder was permanently expelled from school because a condom was found in his bedside locker. There was also a house near the school which was referred to as a brothel because many people came and went. This could have been simply because a large family lived there, I wonder if the owners knew! This was a time when many children born to single mothers and others from 'problem' families were removed from their parents, and sent to Australian orphanages for a better life, which often meant child labour.

I always looked forward to choir, music and Scouts where more personal relationships between staff and pupils could develop. Since these activities were out of choice, motivation was generally high. Being in the chapel choir gave certain privileges, including being able to enter the chapel by a backdoor to put on your cassock. This avoided the risk of punishment by prefects, who inspected us to see if shoes were clean and hair combed. After starting to play the piano, I decided to also learn the viola. To begin with it was difficult as the teacher had no experience of string instruments, and instruction was primarily from books and experimentation.

In my O' level mathematics class, I had consistently done badly in tests and class work until our teacher was changed to Rev. (Daz) White, who was one of the Scout leaders. He went out of his way to explain things to pupils individually. My marks promptly shot up from mediocre to consistently above 95% and this was repeated in the O' level exams themselves. The sciences, for some reason, were not popular subjects but they appealed to me because of the practical components of observation, experiments, nature study and dissection. The teachers of physics and biology were 'gentle' men obviously interested in the subject they taught. Our chemistry teacher however, was always shouting and referring to his teaching manual. In those days formal teacher training was not required and, in retrospect, I think this recent university PhD graduate was somewhat overwhelmed by being put in front of large classes of potentially unruly boys and explosive materials.

English literature classes focused on Shakespeare and poetry and I remember being publicly humiliated once for saying one of my favourite books was 'Swallows and Amazons' by Arthur Ransom. The teacher considered these books to be insufficiently 'imaginative' and not suitable for teenagers. I never understood why, but suspect he had never learnt about the pleasure and thrill of adventure: exploring and observing nature first hand. I was told to stop being childish but this did not increase my motivation to delve more into classical fiction, poetry or Shakespeare. Sadly, I think these classes made me more likely to avoid those sorts of books.

My father removed me from school to complete A' levels at the local higher education college when I was 15. I don't remember being involved in this decision and family financial reasons may have contributed. I saw, by accident, a letter to my father from the headmaster saying this was a disastrous decision. I had mixed emotions: uncertainty about the change, relief from the strict and fearful school atmosphere, but also a sense of excitement. It also allowed me to spend more time on the farm. I was able to keep up friendships with some school colleagues and later hitchhiked around Europe for 2 months with a school friend before going to university.

Higher Education College

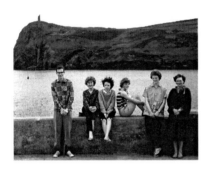

After leaving school early, I studied for 3 A' level exams in college and I feel sure the small classes helped me achieve good results. It was very different from school and we all felt very grown up! Our biology class, shown here, enjoyed a memorable week on the Isle of Man at a marine biology research centre with our caring and enthusiastic teacher, Mrs Byng.

Social life at the college was completely different and I was quite unprepared for my introduction to 'girls'. I was particularly fond of a girl doing a secretarial course and we seemed be getting on very well until we went by bus on a foursome date to see 'Sound of Music' at a cinema in Birmingham. On leaving the cinema, my father, unannounced, was there in the car park to give us all a lift home (not sure why). This promptly killed the romance and it took me ages to recover. I remember overhearing my father say to my mother that 'he should just snap out of it'. Interestingly I later learnt that one of her really nice friends had fancied me throughout the whole episode!

Cubs and Scouts

Throughout junior school I was a Cub and at senior school, a Scout. These organisations gave relief from the 'discipline through fear' atmosphere of school. I found the Cub and Scout leaders inspiring and we learnt many bushcraft skills in a relaxed and friendly team environment. I especially remember my astronomy training which involved lying on the lawn for hours after dark, as well as learning camping skills, and gaining my knitting badge! It is so sad that street lighting in cities now makes it virtually impossible to enjoy star gazing as well as, witnessing the 'Northern Lights' phenomenon.

At one point I was made 'seconder' of the 'Falcons'. However, the patrol leader was one of the biggest school bullies and I later wondered if this was actually a compliment to me that it was thought I might have been able to calm him down. This was not however, a great success, and on a particularly difficult day he told our patrol that we had to let down the tent of one of my best friends. I was the only one in the patrol who had courage to refuse, but we were all taken before the headmaster afterwards for a vigorous telling off and the threat of serious punishment if it happened again. Our scoutmaster, 'Q' Atkin, took me aside afterwards and explained that he knew I had not been involved but did not feel he could separate me out. I appreciated his tactful and reassuring act of diplomacy.

'Q' had been in Greece during the War in very difficult circumstances and I greatly admired him. He introduced us to exploration, survival and coping with the unexpected. Every year there was at least one camp. Once we went to Arisaig, on the West Coast of Scotland, in an old bus that he had renovated. There were no MOTs in those days, and the bus regularly broke down but he was able to mend it, no doubt using his wartime engineering skills. We hiked, biked, swam and climbed. I learnt there is no point in rushing up

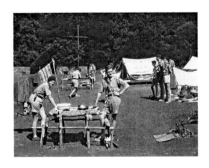

mountains and the secret is to go at a slow steady pace. We also went on trips to Guernsey, Wales, the Lake District and to Austria. Later, after I had left school, 'Q' trained for the church ministry.

One winter challenge was in Wales. After climbing Mount Snowdon, we walked safely through a railway tunnel by carefully studying the train times and having observers at each end to raise the alarm if necessary. This is where I learnt that all tunnels have alcoves at regular intervals in which people can shelter if they were caught out by rapidly approaching trains. I have a feeling that 'Q' had ensured the tunnels were actually out of use, but we did not know that at the time! The picture is of me taking a break during that trip. Sometimes things did go wrong: once we got lost

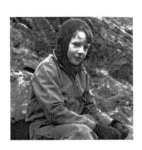

in fog. This tested our map reading skills and we later found that we had been standing on a snow overhang which could easily have broken off, sending us to the valley below. These trips were the culmination of all the skills we had learnt throughout the year: observation, erecting tents, cooking on camp fires, care of equipment, predicting weather, hiking, map reading, scaffolding, bridge building and sending messages through semaphore signals or Morse code.

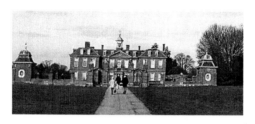

Sometimes small groups of us would youth hostel at weekends and I went on a self-organised hike in Worcestershire to gain my first class badge. We camped in the grounds of Hanbury Hall (above) made famous later by the radio programme 'The Archers'. I still have the logbook I kept at the time. Doing our best, being prepared and self reliance sums up much of what we learnt which contrasts with the newer phenomenon of 'blame culture'.

A Revisit to the School in 2013

What a change! We may complain now about poor school discipline, but surely it is good that teaching now focuses on encouragement rather than threats and intimidation. I sometimes shudder when I hear people say that we should go back to the old methods of education.

I was treated like a VIP for most of the day and given a guided tour by the current headmaster. There are now over 1000 pupils instead of about 400 and while many of the old buildings are still around, there are new science, music, sport and arts centres with superb facilities. There was obviously a relaxed and positive atmosphere between staff and pupils. I shared reminiscences and discussed the changes that had taken place over 60 years. I was told that specifically around the time when I was a pupil, in the 1950s, quite a number of the alumni found their schooldays difficult, which was sort of reassuring. My father had previously taken some 35mm films at a school swimming gala, during some scouting activities and at an annual commemoration day and the current deputy head, with responsibility for school history, was speechless with delight at being given a copy! The headmaster received a jar of my home produced honey.

A highlight of the visit was discovering a very old mulberry tree in a corner of the grounds. It had fascinated me when I was at school because it had magnificent bark, and I knew silk worms could feed off its leaves (although not when grown outdoors in Britain). It had delicious fruits tasting a bit like small loganberries. The headmaster was not aware of its existence but we did some exploration and eventually the head groundsman was able to help us identify it. We found we had actually been within a few feet of it on our previous walk around but the tree was now very much larger! It must have been well over 100 years old and this picture appeared later in the headmaster's school blog.

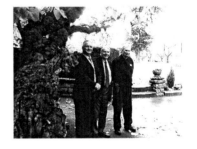

A Gap Year and Exploring Europe

Work on the New M5 Motorway

The M5 motorway was the second motorway to be built in Britain, and during its construction I offered myself as a labourer to earn a bit of money. I think they decided I could add up, so was put into the payroll caravan office, to help work out the wages each week. I cycled the 8 miles each way to work and back. I had a 7am start but this seemed like luxury since my starting time on the dairy farm for milking was 5am.

A high proportion of the labourers were newly arrived immigrants from Pakistan. They were very hard workers and were invariably very friendly and grateful when we went around the sites on a Friday to hand out wage packets, there were no direct transfers to banks in those days.

It was fascinating to witness what goes into make a motorway. This includes the large amount of land needed, a lot more than just the tarmacadam surface. The foundations were very deep with many layers of rock and rubble, and it was important to adjust the camber of the road to allow good drainage. Cuttings and embankments (as on railways) involved big mechanical diggers, unlike days gone by when this was all done by hand. There were many bridges needed, both over and under the motorway, for traffic but also for farm tracks and pedestrians. Then there were all the new signs, motorway cafes and petrol stations as well as opportunities for new tree planting.

The accumulated length of all our tarmacadam roads in the UK is estimated as 350,000 miles. It is only 238,000 miles to go to the moon. We have lost a vast amount of natural land and this surely contributes to the damage now caused by flooding.

Exploring Europe and the Mediterranean Compiled from a Diary I Wrote at the Time

After working on the roads, I joined up with a school friend and we decided to go for an adventure in Europe. We chose a date to leave with no plans other than to cross the English Channel and take it from there. We had rucksacks, a tent and about £100 in cash each (about £1000 in 2010). We were both a bit nervous but excited. On the day before we left, I went to an evensong service at our local church and to my surprise the vicar included a prayer for those leaving home.

I was not aware of my parents being concerned, although in retrospect, I think my mother had been anxious. My adventures while Scouting had probably given them some reassurance that we would be able to look after ourselves sensibly. It must be remembered that in those days there were no reliable telephones, mobile phones or emails. We could not receive letters but I sent back regular postcards. I wonder how many parents now would take such a relaxed approach.

Hitchhiking Techniques and Experiences

In those days, hitchhiking (known as 'auto-stop' on the continent), was not seen to be particularly risky and we soon learnt the tricks of the trade about where to stand when looking for lifts. Most of those who offered lifts were very friendly and helpful, often going out of their way to drop us off in convenient places and provide us with snacks and friendly banter. We were told in advance that having a Union Jack displayed on our rucksacks might help us to get lifts. I think because this said to drivers that we were genuine explorers, and not simply looking for a lift home after missing the bus or having had too much to drink! It also implied that our native language was English, which we found encouraged some to practice their language skills on us, the exception being in France, where English is less enthusiastically embraced. Many drivers seemed to give us lifts because we looked young and 'innocent' and they genuinely wanted to be helpful. A few drivers asked for payment, but we politely turned down their offers despite some being persistent.

Each morning we decided where we might go that day, and if we liked a place we could stay for several days. It was a rare freedom from any sort of planning. Nowadays I find I prefer to get things planned in advance because of other commitments, time constraints and budgeting. We often stayed in youth hostels but having a tent meant if we were stuck we just had to find somewhere to pitch it. We used the European Youth Hostellers' Guide. This was before the days of the 'Lonely Planet' series of books which has recently acquired a 'biblical' reputation for backpackers. Our International Student's Card allowed us free into many museums, art galleries and archeological sites.

We were never aware of formal campsites, which are mostly now designed for campers with cars or camper vans. When we camped, we usually chose somewhere near the roadside or in a park. Once when it was very late and dark in Switzerland, we went through a hole in a hedge and pitched our tent only to find in the morning we had camped in the grounds of a very smart mansion. Fortunately the gardener was very friendly, and even brought us some milk for our breakfast.

Places we visited

The following is based on a simple diary I kept during the trip. We stayed for some time in Greece, where the diary took second place, and I have to rely mostly on memory.

France

We nearly missed the boat from Dover and there were only a few regular ferries in those days. There were no hovercraft or ships designed for juggernaut lorries. We arrived in Calais at about midday, ate our sandwiches supplied from home, and after getting advice from a friendly Italian

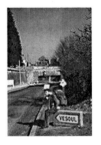

man (who clearly enjoyed his wine), found the road out to Vesoul. We hitched to Boulogne where we stayed in the local hostel. A useful tip we learnt quickly was to stay in one place suitable for vehicles to stop easily while hitching lifts and not to keep walking.

The next morning we got a lift with a very friendly driver in a fish lorry heading inland, from Boulogne to Arras, with his catch of the day. This was followed by luxury transport in a very comfortable lorry with a less smelly cargo (although the fish aroma was not unpleasant) going from Holland to Paris.

We arrived in Paris at about 11pm and with difficulty found a hostel, which was a converted toilet in the middle of a boulevard, that turned out to be a refuge for heavy drinkers. We moved the next day to a more distant but quieter place in the Pigalle district. Our student cards allowed us free bus and underground journeys which was useful because the Louvre, Notre Dame Cathedral, Montmartre and Napoleon's mausoleum were very spread out. The metro was efficient but when the doors shut they did so very suddenly and with a lot of noise! We climbed on foot all the way up the Eiffel Tower; I don't think this is now allowed and you have to go by lift for the final ascent. On one occasion, we were stopped by armed gendarmes to see if we were carrying any weapons. This was not done in a threatening manner and I think they had nothing better to do at the time. A highlight was breakfast in street side cafes with freshly baked French bread and coffee!

Getting lifts out of Paris was difficult since we had to travel quite a long way to first establish ourselves on the correct N-9 highway heading for Switzerland. Arriving quite late in Troyes, we found the hostel was shut so we slept the night in a cowshed with the agreement of a kind farmer. The cows kept us warm since it was freezing outside, but there was fresh warm milk in the morning. The next day we went to Belfort where the youth hostel was first rate, and the supper was excellent. En route, we admired buzzards and much mistletoe in the many fruit orchards. Most fellow hostellers were French, and I was pleasantly surprised to find how useful my schoolboy French was and how quickly having to speak in a foreign language improves fluency.

Switzerland

Our final lift to Switzerland was with an inebriated Englishman who spent a lot of time telling us about his experiences in both World Wars. I wrote a postcard home in the car but after crossing into Basel I realized the stamp was French so I was allowed back across the border briefly to find a postbox. It was March so there was still plenty of snow but the hostel was good and even had a television! We purchased a detailed RAC road map of Europe which proved invaluable for the rest of our adventure. Youth hostels in Switzerland were very clean, well-organised and everyone spoke English.

From Basle we took a bus then steamboat to Zurich where we got in touch with a medical friend of my father. He put us up for a couple of nights in his home, where we were made very welcome. He took us exploring with him, including a visit to his medical school. For some reason I remember a special spaghetti with tomato sauce and cheese that his wife made for us! We took a train up the local Üetliberg Mountain followed by an evening out exploring the nightlife of beer cellars and coffee bars which made us feel very grown-up! On leaving Zurich, I felt seriously homesick for a while, related I am sure to our few days of relaxation and comfort in Dr Freihofer's home.

Next stop was Altdorf which is best known as the place where William Tell is said to have shot an apple off his son's head. The town is at altitude, a typical house is shown. We 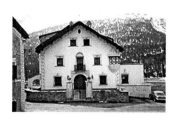 experienced fishing through holes in ice on the lake (it was still winter) and ringing a cowbell to summon a boat to take us to an island restaurant. We met several husky mountain rescue dogs and learnt that dogs are not simply pets and rat catchers.

Italy (and a brief return to France)
Our first stop was Milan and this was the first time we found language a problem since few spoke English or French. Also, there were no cooking facilities in the rather expensive hostel and it was so we went on the next day to Turin on the way to explore the French Riviera. This meant going back over the

Southern Alps where, to our surprise, there was more snow than in Switzerland and one of our lifts resulted in a number of skids going down icy steep roads but the driver seemed very used to this. Turin is a substantial city but was very different from the more industrial Milan. There was still no food in the hostel so we ate in a student refectory.

Nice gave us our first glimpse of the Mediterranean with palm trees, orange groves and a warm but wet climate. We learnt about 'tourist prices' and so ate in back streets. My main 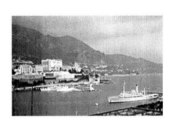 memory of Nice was of wealth: with the promenade, luxury yachts, heavy traffic and expensive seafood. One day, we caught a bus to Monaco where we needed our passports to enter since it is an independent principality and then walked back along the coast.

Pisa and Florence

We had to quickly learn that in Italy it was common practice to try to take tourists, including students, 'for a ride' when

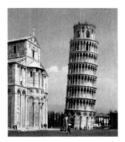 it comes to prices.

The leaning tower of Pisa is part of a church complex and leans by about 4.5 metres at the top. The inside is full of supporting pillars and internal scaffolding to keep it upright. The hostel

in Pisa was being renovated, but temporary accommodation was available in an adapted stable.

Florence allowed us to begin to get an insight into Italian art and history. The Ponte-de-Vechio bridge is certainly nostalgic and gave a feel for the past except that we found it was lined with tourist shops, rather than markets for locals. The day we left Florence there was heavy rain and we had learned it was more difficult to get lifts when you and your rucksacks are drenched, so we took a bus along the coast road to Rome.

Rome

Rome was very busy but nothing like compared with now. Getting around involved lots of walking and even then, lives seemed to be at risk trying to get across the huge roundabout that surrounds the Colosseum! Rome was our introduction to having to cope with constant approaches of vendors asking for money in exchange for (often) frivolous tourist souvenirs.

The Vatican must be a 'one and only' with all its history, the many buildings, the cathedral and its obvious wealth combined with religious history. I was interested in the emergency escape route, if needed, along the inside of a wall leading to the river. I was disappointed to find very

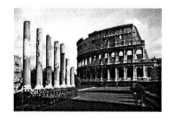

touristy items being sold inside the cathedral. The many smaller, unrelated churches around the city were an interesting contrast and usually very ornate. Rome itself, a bit like Paris, was very memorable but I tended to prefer the 'out of town' sites we visited including the famous water aqueduct.

Naples and Capri

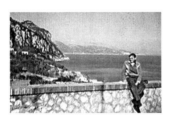

There were dramatic views from our hostel which was on the hills to the north of the city. There was another less salubrious hostel in the city. We ate well on fruit and pastas. The pasta is such a versatile dish and included many more varieties than was available in Britain, but the pasta had to be fresh not dried!

Naples was very different from Rome with less traffic, a slower pace of life and more obvious poverty. Prostitution was common, especially in the dock areas, and young male tourists seemed to be targeted. The Pompeii ruins were only partially excavated and could be explored fully in an afternoon. Herculaneum is smaller and better preserved, with several multistoried houses and impressive under-floor, wood-fired central heating.

Capri has a very island atmosphere dominated by proximity to the sea and with many gardens and luxury houses. A boat trip to a less than impressive sea cave was spoilt by the boat owner refusing at the entrance to take us inside unless we paid extra money on top of what we had already paid for the trip!

Travel from Naples to Greece by Sea

The journey lasted about 24 hours overnight on a cargo boat. We took our own sandwiches and drinks and were offered bunks in a very stuffy, hot and airless cabin but preferred to stay on deck. We settled down on the deck and later slept in a lifeboat. We were rewarded by a dramatic view of Mount Etna as we passed Sicily. This was the first time I had seen an active volcano and was very surprised to see snow on its summit.

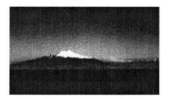

Arriving in Piraeus, tired and dirty, the sight greeting us was queues of sailors, and we only realized afterwards they were waiting to enter the local brothel.

Greece: Athens

After exploring many of the archeological sites we separated to spend a fortnight with separate Greek families to help their children practice speaking English. This was arranged for us by an Englishman living in Athens who was a friend of my farming mentor, Ed Hall's cousin, these days this might be called 'networking', but I would prefer to simply say 'friendliness'.

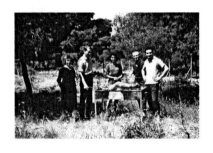

The family had some land where they had orange and olive trees. The flavor of fully ripe oranges picked straight from the tree has forever spoilt any enjoyment I get from eating oranges we get in the UK - picked unripe and rarely fully sweetened in the sun.

One evening, on the way home to the family, I was caught up in a riot. I had the unpleasant experience of being sprayed with tear gas when I accidentally went the wrong way down a street and met the riot police coming in the opposite direction! My hosts said, 'this happens all the time' due to the hot weather and the excitable Greek temperament.

Mykonos

We the had a marvellously relaxing 2 weeks camping on a deserted beach and it was a long time before the island became converted into a popular tourist resort. Despite not being able to converse with local villagers, a family befriended us and their daughter volunteered to wash our dirty clothes together with their own on a scrubbing stone in small stream near our campsite. The sea food in dockside restaurants was memorable, as

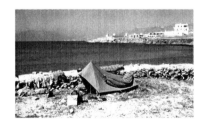

was the Retsina wine and
Ouzo spirit which was
said to make you go blind
if drunk to excess!

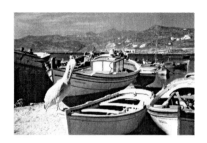

There was a local pelican
living in the harbour and
no doubt well fed.

The beach by our campsite is now a resort with numerous
modern hotels, bars, discos, deck chairs and parasols.

Yugoslavia

This was our first experience of a communist country.
Everything was very basic and the pace of life slow. A
short trip is not an opportunity to really get to know and
understand lifestyles but there was none of the natural,
sometimes annoying, friendliness we met in Italy and Greece.
Orange squash was produced by just one manufacturer and
seemed to be mostly chemicals, with little orange flavour.
The choice of foods generally was very limited. We learnt
about mixed-sex toilets where men enter from one side of
the street and women from the other to meet underground in
the middle around a large hole in the ground. I felt that this
rather sad picture was mainly a town phenomenon and not
so obvious in the country where we could get fresh orange
juice and the villagers seemed more naturally friendly.

One of our lifts was with a cheery driver with whom we could

successfully communicate using
body language alone. Finally in
Dubrovnik we were given a lift
by an obviously well-off English
man with an open top sports car
who drove us about 200 miles
from Dubrovnik to Trieste.

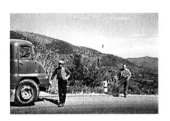

Back to Italy: Venice

Venice is unique and the lack of motor traffic once you cross
the bridge from the station is special. Architecturally there
were comparisons with the ancient crannogs in Scotland
where residences were based on stilts driven into the beds
of lochs taking advantage of the fact that wood kept per-
manently wet and deprived of oxygen does not normally
rot. We learned about Venice's historical role in international travel and trade: visiting the island where travellers
and immigrants were examined and quarantined. I felt
fascinated more with the ambiance, than the tourist sites,
maybe coloured by our stay being short and interrupted by
a bout of traveller's diarrhoea. When there was no room
available in the youth hostel, the canal had to act as a toilet
and I don't think we were the only people to use it in this
way.

By this time we were both feeling ready to return home and,
as it turned out, our final journey from Venice was with a
lovely couple from Holland and their 2 daughters. We were
wined, dined and they paid for accommodation for us in a

smart hotel as we travelled with them to link with a train to Calais and home. This was a relaxing final journey without having to make decisions on routes and food or which sites to visit.

Return home

The White Cliffs of Dover were a memorable sight, and today travellers will miss this experience when arriving home by plane or through the channel tunnel. Although our feelings can hardly be compared to those of the soldiers being evacuated in desperate straits from Dunkirk at the start of World War II. Our first stop in Dover was a café where the waitress called us 'dear', this was very moving because by that time we were very ready to get home.

The final leg of our adventure was by train, and my mother came to pick us up from the railway station. She was so excited, that on exiting the car park, she drove the wrong way around a roundabout.

MEDICAL SCHOOL
AND A RESTLESS SPIRIT

My Uncle Eric had told me that university was one third study, one third learning about life and one third fun. I tried to take this advice with me and avoid being 'just a medical student'. With this in mind, I chose on his advice to stay in a university hall of residence called Manor House, which was an adapted mansion that had previously belonged to the Cadbury family of chocolate fame. It was in a quiet area, 3 miles from the University with extensive grounds: large lawns, a forested area, walled garden and tennis courts. There was also a lake, which had been commissioned by the Cadbury family as a philanthropic venture, to give employment to people during the recession of the 1930s. It was stimulating to be able to mix with students studying a wide range of subjects, unlike many medical students who chose the independence of their own flats. This normally meant their closest friends were all 'medics'.

The oldest part of the house contained a number of study bedrooms, a lounge, dining room and an indoor games room. There was also a modern bed and study room extension. Upstairs in the old house, there was an original Victorian toilet positioned at the far the end of a 5 metre long narrow room with a superb florally decorated toilet basin. I wonder what has happened to it and whether someone who eventually thought it too old fashioned has sadly destroyed it. The house and grounds have sadly now been bought over for development. The whole area is 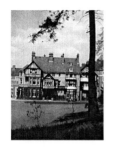 a large housing estate and most of the trees, pond and lawns have gone.

Each evening there was formal dinner at a fixed time. A bell summoned us and we were expected to be smartly dressed. There was waitress service and a high table where students took it in turns to eat with the resident university staff and principal. Once a year there was a formal dinner and ball arranged by the student committee and once I invited Ed Hall from my farming days to come along as a guest. He invited Noreen, a teacher at a local school, whom he later married. Ed lived into his 80s and I still keep in touch with Noreen.

The length of time students could stay in Manor House was normally 2 years, but if you were elected onto the student committee then you could stay longer. So I became bar and darts club treasurer and stayed for 4 years. During this time I won a competition for the fastest drinker of a pint of beer! During university holidays only medical students were still around so we all stayed in the old house. This always seemed a special time.

One initiative I started up was a discussion club, which we held in the principal's rooms. We chose a topic to debate in turns and enjoyed the principal's hospitality including snacks and some of his wine while we tried to solve the world's problems. This was when the Soviet Union and the West were stockpiling huge arsenals of nuclear weapons. The Vietnam War had started and then there was John Kennedy's assassination and the Cuban missile crisis. Stimulated by these events, peace movements sprung up particularly among the young. This was the age of 'hippies' and the 'flower people' who wanted to demonstrate that there could be an alternative to continual conflict - lessons humanity still does not seem to have learnt.

Medical School

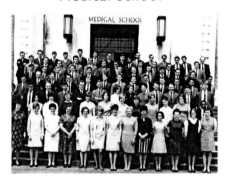

My intake year at medical school (shown) consisted of about 70% male and 30% female students. This proportion has now been reversed in most medical schools and so more medical students need to be trained, as many female doctors later choose to work part-time when childbearing and caring for young children. We studied non-clinical subjects such anatomy, physiology and pharmacology for the first two years. These consisted of lectures, human dissection and laboratory classes.

Pre-clinical Years

These 2 years were dominated by anatomy in the first year and physiology in the second year. I was fascinated by embryology which showed how we could trace human evolution through various stages of development right back to the fish. For example, we sometimes develop branchial cysts in our neck that are thought to be remnants of gills used for breathing under water. I did well in anatomy but less so in physiology possibly due, I think, to a poor intro-duction to organic chemistry at school.

We also started to learn about pharmacology, pathology and statistics. Statistical analysis was done by hand using squared paper to display records, making up our own graphs and sometimes using 'punch cards' with a knitting needle to sort out data with particular characteristics such as male from female, different ages and so on. Computers were very much in their infancy and experimental: the medical school had one which occupied a whole small room. This was well before the days of silicon chips on which vast amounts of data can be stored, and which led to the advent of the small personal computer. The only exam I failed at medical school was statistics, but it was not in the main curriculum so did not need to be repeated. Later on, I developed a real interest on epidemiology but have always sought advice if any study I was involved in required complicated statistical analysis. The term 'social medicine' which we were introduced to has gone through many transitions since and included what we now call 'preventive medicine', 'occupational' and 'public' health. Part of our experience included visiting factories and going down a coal mine. This was the time when the associations between smoking and lung cancer, between coal dust and pneumoconiosis, and the dangers of asbestos were being recognised. A major achievement in Birmingham was showing clearly through archived records that the decline in tuberculosis in the UK had begun long before the introduction of effective antituberculosis treatment and was related to improvements in housing, hygiene and to some extent diet. Legislation requiring 'Don't spit or you will be prosecuted' notices on public transport was introduced to try and cut down its spread.

At the end of pre-clinical years, like many medical students, I became a bit restless and requested time off to 'go around the world'. This request was politely refused by the Dean. However, later I was chosen to spend 3 months in Africa on a final year student exchange scheme studying in Harare, so I don't think the Dean had forgotten my interest in travel and exploration. The African experience, described later, made me very aware that health was not simply the absence of disease: lifestyles, attitudes, preventing illness and how we relate to our environment are so important.

Clinical Years

These 3 years were spent mostly in hospital where we were allocated in small groups to most of the main specialities, with one formal lecture in late afternoons. The currently popular student selected modules and electives did not exist.

On our 4 month rotating ward attachments, we were individually allocated patients to clerk in and follow-up during their stay. My first patient had a thoracic aortic aneurism and was otherwise a fit man, but he died on the operating table due to bleeding which was very distressing for all involved. This was my first experience of seeing someone die and for many medical students early clinical years were the first opportunity to experience death first-hand. I was very familiar with these life events in birds and animals from my rural and farming background, but this was a new experience.

A major source of our knowledge and understanding of these events came from the very experienced ward sisters, who saw guiding both medical and nursing students, as part of a long-term career. At this time most did not choose to enter more highly paid administration roles, as is now common. They were strict but in a way that gained respect from both junior nurses and other staff. Many lived per-manently in the hospital and the majority were unmarried. Likewise, it was obligatory for junior student nurses to live in the nurses home, which was strictly out of bounds for medical students!

I enjoyed my obstetrics placement in a small maternity hospital where my first delivery experience was with an Irish woman, pregnant for the eighth time. She told me to go to bed after I had sat up with her until 2am and that she would call me. She did call, but I was too late since her delivery took only 5 minutes - she was very experienced.

She was very upset and apologetic, and insisted on giving me a box of chocolates.

Learning from patients themselves during clinical attachments seemed to me to have similarities with farming: with its focus on working with nature rather than seeing ourselves as detached or superior. During our paediatric placements we were allocated to a child and were expected to relate to their family as well. Most of us visited the child and family on one or two occasions at home after discharge. These visits were our only exposure to general practice during our training. This lack of general practice exposure led many to think that a future career outside hospital was in some way a second rate career option, or even a sign of 'failure'. It was not surprising that those that organised the curricula were exclusively hospital based.

There was also no clinical infectious disease teaching, only microbiology from a laboratory perspective. Later, when I undertook general practice locums, I had to teach myself from textbooks since a high proportion of new consultations were, and still are, due to infection. In the 1960s measles, mumps, whooping cough, rubella and scarlet fever for example, were still common place.

Something that has changed since, is that we were allowed and encouraged in our final year, to undertake locums for junior qualified doctors. These optional placements were not regulated and the amount of supervision was very variable. It was usually the registrars to whom we were responsible. Not everyone undertook these but I did several and they were a good introduction for what was to come during our first postgraduate hospital appointments. Sometimes they proved useful when it came to applying for junior appointments which was done on an individual application basis with the consultant concerned, and not through a formal allocation process which came later.

At medical school, music and a lot of other activities like sport, tended to take a back seat. Study was intensive and one friend, who spent a lot of time in the university choir, failed all his exams after 2nd year and had to leave. There was however, a hospital Gilbert and Sullivan group that I joined. Once, during the opera Pirates of Penzance, I forgot to put my pirates hat back on after the interval, which was very embarrassing, but I don't think many noticed!

Having been involved in teaching throughout my later career, my impression is that students now come to medical school much better prepared academically than we were, but may take longer after qualifying to gain confidence in clinical decision-making. At school they also now seem to get more useful opportunities to debate, reflect and undertake written and presentation skills. Although, their handwriting is awful since in these days of computers they get little practice! However computers are an advantage when it comes to undertaking projects and assignments: allowing quick access to a wide range of publications without spending time searching through library shelves and the old 'Index Medicus' books for information and references. I think students are also much more aware of global health issues for the same reason and therefore, think much more broadly when it comes to career choices.

Student Exchange at Harare Medical School, Rhodesia (now Zimbabwe) 1965

This was different from the current elective schemes for medical students. It was a formal exchange of four final year students from Birmingham with medical students from Harare, and the time counted fully towards our formal medical education. At the time, Birmingham was helping set up the first medical school and teaching hospital in Rhodesia, and doctors and nurses from Birmingham went out on temporary contracts to fill senior clinical and teaching posts.

It was a very formative time and probably the trigger for my future interest in working abroad, contributing to healthcare in poorer countries and learning about different cultures. Perhaps I was also seeking to follow the compassionate and philanthropic example of my Uncle Eric.

The journey out was special because it involved travelling on a VC10 jet aircraft, the first jet aircraft introduced into commercial passenger service in the 1960s. The plane had to stop in West Africa to refuel and went on to Johannesburg where we transferred into a propellor driven Viscount Valiant for the final leg to Harare. These smooth, stable and quieter turboprop engines now tend to be seen as old fashioned and only used for short flights in smaller aircraft. During the 1950s they replaced the noisy valve and piston driven engines used in military aircraft extensively during World War II.

There were two main native African tribes in Rhodesia: the Mashona and Matabele. The Matabele were said to be peace-loving and Matabele the warriors, but I could not tell any personality differences in those Africans I met.

I developed a great respect for the senior consultant in Harare, Professor Gelfand who had lived all his life in Southern Africa. He had enormous personal experience of African culture and traditions and had written widely on traditional African medical practices. This included papers on widespread killer diseases such as malaria, trypanosomiasis and schistosomiasis and traditional healing practices such as making several parallel cuts in the skin over the site of pain or 'ringing' with a hot tin or metal cup, when it was thought the burn and residual scar would release evil spirits or imagined poisons.

We stayed in good accommodation in the hospital and ward rounds lasted about eight hours from early morning till the evening. The Professor would undertake procedures like lumbar and cervical spinal taps during the rounds. These were often needed urgently because of the high incidence of meningitis, particularly due to tuberculosis. He introduced us to the importance of data collection and epidemiology and would repeatedly say 'Sister, please bring me

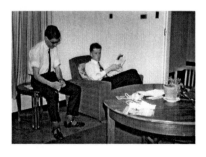 my typhoid book' or 'my schistosomiasis book' or 'my snake bite book'. These simple records were kept on a special shelf at the end of each ward and he would jot

down important data that later provided a wealth of information for research and improving disease management. We were there during the civil war before Rhodesia became independent when the country was renamed Zimbabwe to relate to its historical past. This meant we saw patients in the emergency department with wounds and injuries of various types. Excessive alcohol drinking was a common problem usually from drinking local home made brews which, especially in the malnourished, could lead to delirium tremens with violent and uncontrolled behaviour. Intravenous 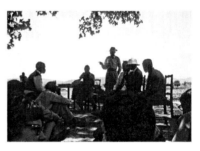 multivitamins seemed to quickly control the paranoia.

We went on trips to villages where we learnt first hand about local cultural practices (photo above of a village elders meeting). Some of these trips lasted for several days and involved collecting data for simple but valuable research studies. For example, recording splenomegaly was a simple 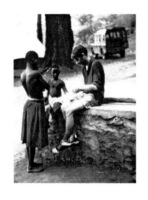 way of estimating the prevalence of malaria in an area where malaria was the most common cause. Immediate action, as well as future planning, could be taken such as giving advice on eliminating mosquito breeding sites, using mosquito nets and spraying houses with insecticide. This picture is of me treating a child bitten by a night adder.

Goiters due to iodine deficiency were very common in certain areas and one of the medical registrars, Hilton Whittle, whom I had known when he 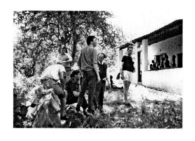 was a Birmingham medical student (standing in the middle looking towards the clinic), arranged an expedition to find out the incidence in an area known to have the problem. This allowed us to identify and explain the need for iodine supplements and resulted in my first medical 'publication' when Hilton, unexpectedly and after I had returned to the UK, insisted I should be a co-author. Since then I have been very aware of the importance of involving junior doctors in research and any related publications wherever this is appropriate. This insight has been relevant later both in India and in the UK.

Multiple wives were common especially for village chiefs and the wealthier. It is apparently still the case in many parts that a man will marry only after his prospective bride has proven she is able to become pregnant. Multiple sexual relationships were normal and it is no surprise that in this setting HIV infection has become such a serious problem. Education was a luxury only for the few so trying to explain, for example, how infections spread was extremely difficult. We learned about subsistence living which is not as bad (except for the destitute) as some from consumer societies may think. We joined discussions about medical problems and sat in on 'community council' meetings. At these meetings the elders of the village arbitrated on disputes between neighbours, divorces and other local issues, usually outside and often under a banyan tree.

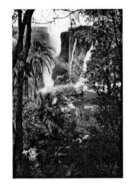 On a short holiday trip to Victoria Falls, I had set off to walk over a railway bridge that crosses the river. I had been told the falls were more impressive from the northern bank and I was keen to take a photograph. In my naivety I had forgotten that the river was effectively the Rhodesia - Zambian border and this was during the Rhodesian Civil War of Independence. After a phone call to his superior, the very pleasant guard kindly conducted me at gunpoint to take my photograph, which I treasure, and wished me well when I set of to walk back across the bridge.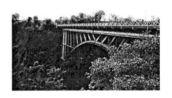

On a weekend break after hiring a car and driving through Mozambique to Beira on the coast of the Indian Ocean, we stayed in a beach hut and swam in the sea one evening after dark. On return I entered the hut, switched on the light, and was thrown across the room by an electric shock maybe made worse by my wet feet and wearing no shoes. Could have been worse … !

I found my introduction to the Rhodesian form of apartheid very emotionally distressing. I found it difficult to accept that it was a crime to go out for a drink to the same bar as African student friends simply because of the colour of their skin. Adult servants in the houses were called house or garden 'boys' and it was strange to see elderly men and women treated as children. They were normally treated well with affection but they could not be allowed to step out of line and small misdemeanors could promptly mean dismissal. This discrimination came home to me again when we went to have a meal at a restaurant during one of our expeditions and the African colleagues who were helping us collect blood samples were not allowed in. I refused the meal and went for a walk on my own to the consternation of my student companions who feared for my safety. Within the hospital where the rules were less closely observed, I became friends with one of the African nurses who shared her concerns about her father who was in jail for being a member of the African National Council. The ANC was

seeking racial equality but it had been outlawed as a terrorist group. On a lighter note, she introduced me to some of the history of Southern Africa and fasci- 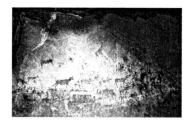 nating prehistoric rock paintings created by her ancestors.

When returning to the UK, I had to spend a night in Johannesburg. I exited the airport through a door behind some left-luggage lockers but was escorted back by an armed white policeman and told firmly I had used the 'blacks only' door. This was a punishable crime so I had to use the large glass fronted main door that was reserved for 'whites'. It is sad to see there are still many examples of 'racism' although not always related to skin colour but under the guise of castes, tribes and radical political and bigoted religious groups.

Short Holiday Trips While at Medical School

Paris

I was able to revisit some places I had seen during my European hitchhiking adventure and I enjoyed the quiet and the relaxed atmosphere, which the French seem to encourage. Walking along the River Seine was a highlight as well as visiting Notre Dame Cathedral that encouraged me to read Victor Hugo's book, 'The Hunchback of Notre Dame'. Later I enjoyed 'Les Miserables' even more, which I have read from cover to cover on several occasions, usually when on holiday. The combination of adventure with survival, despite injustice and poverty, combined with a very real and spiritual description of the potential of unconditional love, I continue to find gripping and inspiring. Beware it is a very long read and there are lots of philosophical interludes!

During this trip, I found myself accidentally staying in a Bordello in the Sorbonne. It combined as a guesthouse, which is something I have also noticed in India, and I suspect is more common than many think.

Gibraltar and Morocco

During this short trip, I stayed in a 'Toc H' hostel that

was very comfortable and had a rooftop balcony ideal for relaxing and reading without disturbance. By this time I was interested in Ernest Hemingway's books mainly because he had been a medical student. This trip was on a very tight budget and my first night, after arriving late by plane, was spent in a small derelict electrical transmission shed near a lighthouse and next to a rainwater collection area, which stored drinking water in an underground 'lake'.

To spend a few days in Morocco I had to cross the Straits of Gibraltar to Tangiers and the first uncomfortable thing I experienced on arrival was being asked to buy hashish. I took a train and then a bus to Fez - an inland town with fascinating traditional architecture and a history of being a university centre for studying Islam.

My first night in Fez was spent in very basic accommodation in the old town or Casbah where the only washing facility was a trough in a central courtyard and the toilet was a communal bucket. During the night I was woken by a lot of scratching and rustling so I put on my torch to find several large rats running about the small cubical. When they entered under the door there was a scrape as the hinges were lifted and then a clump as the door dropped back into place. I threw my shoes at them and they went out the same way. I am surprised I did not end up with bedbugs but I did get out alive! The next morning, to recover, I went to a more modern part of the town where I knocked on the door of a church manse and spent the next night in luxury being looked after by the minister and his wife. It all added up to be a memorable, if not wholly enjoyable, experience culminating in being propositioned, as a young naïve male, by an English businessman on the train back to Tangiers who offered me free accommodation for the night which I discovered later was intended to be in a double bed. I managed to quickly escape and get the next ferry back to Gibraltar.

Italy

My return trip to Italy was much more relaxed. A friend from medical school had been asked to deliver a car to a friend of his father in Naples who paid all our expenses including a train trip back to the UK. This meant we had, more or less, control over our travel plans and could live in 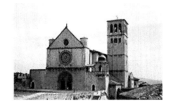 relative luxury visiting Milan, Florence and Rome on the way. A highlight was time spent in Assisi where I began to learn about the history and teachings of St Francis. His simple living in close proximity to nature interested me as well as his quote: 'The responsibility of man is to protect and enjoy nature as stewards of God's creation because we are creatures ourselves'. The basilica of St Francis is shown here.

The Hebridean Islands

With a student friend, John Aldridge, in our final year, I went for a short camping trip to explore the Scottish Hebridean Islands which we had not visited before. We took the train to Ullapool and then the ferry overnight to Lewis, before hitch-hiking our way down to the South Uist Islands and Barra. Finally we crossed over to Mull and Iona before going back to the mainland.

At a youth dance in Stornaway, the capital of Lewis, on the Saturday night, it was difficult to see in the room because of smoke, smoking at that time was clearly meant to show you were 'cool' - this word only came into common parlance many years later to replace being 'with it'!

Lewis, at that time, had very strict 'no work on Sundays' rules and there were no buses, very few cars on the road and no shops open. We were the only people in the little hotel we stayed at and had to make our own breakfast since the staff were not allowed to work. We then attended a local 'wee free' church service which included an hour long sermon full of 'fire and brimstone'.

Remembering that this was at the height of the Cold War, it was interesting to see from a distance the testing site for long-range missiles on Benbecula. Testing no longer takes place here but there is still a radar tracking station surveying the East Atlantic Ocean and the land mass of Scotland.

Many short ferry trips were involved through Skye to Mallaig (right), then to Oban and Mull until we arrived in Iona (over page) where we camped on the beach by the Abbey only to find water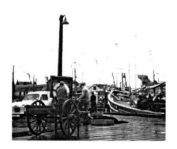

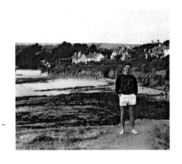

lapping our sleeping bags during the night - we had not realised that because there was a full moon there was going to be a high tide! Visiting Staffa to see Fingal's cave made famous by Mendelssohn's Hebridean overture was a highlight.

Pre-registration Surgical and Medical Appointments (1966-67)

A 'pre-registration year' is an accurate description of our first year after qualifying since we were not formally registered doctors although this was never actually explained to us at the time. My first post combined general surgery and ortho-paedics in, what was then called, East Birmingham Hospital - now called Heartlands. It had a more relaxed atmosphere than the more formal teaching hospitals. However we were expected to be competent doctors and had to take on a lot of responsibility. I was frequently left on my own on-call at nights and weekends with cover only by a senior registrar from his home. The value of having done some student locum placements was clear. I was the only house officer on the team and so had the advantage of much personal teaching from the senior registrar and consultant.

I developed the valuable habit of after admitting patients, when I had a spare moment either in my room or on the ward, reading up about their signs, symptoms and likely differential diagnoses. The classic book 'Hutchinson's Clinical Methods' was invaluable and in the 1960s it was the history and examination that were paramount in making a diagnosis since immediate laboratory tests were usually limited to haemoglobin, white blood cell counts, urea and electrolytes and serum amylase. There were no ultrasound or scanning facilities. We performed urine microscopy and erythrocyte sedimentation rates on the ward ourselves. I became competent in procedures like venous infusions, lumbar punctures, chest drains and abdominal paracentesis and removed appendixes under supervision.

My second pre-registration post in general medicine and diabetes was at the General Hospital in Birmingham. This was very valuable experience but since it was a teaching hospital we were still seen and treated as students, so discouraged from making any decisions without consulting the on-call registrar. Since I had become used to taking on responsibilities myself, I got into trouble in my first week for treating a patient who was in a diabetic coma - the patient I am pleased to say recovered quickly!

One interesting link with my time in Africa when a patient complained of recurrent abdominal pain and blood in his urine. He had previously undergone a variety of invasive diagnostic procedures and even had a blood transfusion when a lot of blood was found in his urine bottle. I got chatting to him one evening about Rhodesia where he said he had been, and he mentioned seeing elephants in the Wankie Game Reserve from the road, while travelling to Victoria Falls. I knew the game Reserve was not near the main road and he turned out to have been putting animal blood into his urine to attract doctor's attention - a classic case of Munchausan's syndrome.

The workload this time was 6 days a week and 24 hours a day and involved between 15-20 admissions every third day when on call. Working throughout the day and night meant that we looked after our own patients right through their hospital stay which is something that rota systems now make impossible. In addition we did duties in the casualty department on three evenings a week and one weekend in two. This would have been impossible safely without continual advice and supervision from the very experienced casualty nursing sisters. There were no such things as formal protocols and procedures for managing patients as there are now.

A strong community spirit developed in the doctor's mess where we had our bedrooms and were cared for in a very motherly fashion by the domestic staff who would bring cups of tea in the morning and make us something fresh to eat at any time of day or night. Christmas always involved a special party where we would dress up and make fun of our seniors on stage. A consultant's small sports car was once dragged up steps onto the roof of the hospital to everyone's amusement.

Overall during my house jobs, I lost 1½ stone in weight in 12 months but the experience gained was special and stood us in good stead. I don't think I would like to go through this exhausting experience again but we learned an enormous amount about clinical care in a very short period of time. It is thought that current pre-registration posts are much less strenuous but I don't think this is always the case and it varies between hospitals. There is also a lot more involved now with the advent of high-tech emergency and intensive care, procedures and protocols and arranging more complicated investigations.

For those training now, it must be very difficult to imagine what is was like before all this technology was available. We did not even have 'pagers' or mobile phones so trying to contact a doctor meant a combination of phone calls between wards and outpatients or sending someone from the ward to find you. On the positive side, however, it meant we spent more time actually on the wards with patients where there was usually a rest room and also saw our patients repeatedly during the day and of special value was the regular late evening ward round.

A SABBATICAL YEAR IN CAMBRIDGE AND MY INTRODUCTION TO GENERAL PRACTICE

At medical school the formal teaching focused almost exclusively on disease diagnosis, treatment and management. Ecological, spiritual, religious and moral aspects of health I can only remember once being mentioned, and that was during an explanation about the symptoms of schizophrenia. Health in its broader personal and community sense was largely ignored except by a few of our teachers - perhaps for me the most influential was the consultant physician I worked for during my second-registration house job. He was very knowledgeable, thoughtful and compassionate and was one of those physicians who spoke with gentle authority that gained respect. When I told him I was thinking of undertaking a sabbatical year to study health and philosophy, he was one of the very few who did not think I had 'lost my senses'!

Also we were taught how important it was for medicine to be based on sound scientific studies (now called 'evidence based' medicine) but no one ever explained what science was except in terms of research. I was frustrated because I felt that medical practice required more than using simply a drug or surgery-based approach to managing disease, important as these are.

Westminster College, Cambridge

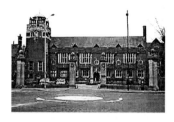

This is a theological college affiliated to the University. It is residential with a mix of students including undergraduates studying a wide variety of subjects (something like Manor House), those on a sabbatical year like myself who were from the UK, or overseas and postgraduates undertaking research or training for the church ministry. It respected Cambridge University traditions such as allocation of personal tutors and advisors, formal meals for staff and students with the wearing of gowns, daily chapel services and weekly round table evening discussions lead by both staff and students in turn on topics not necessarily related to the students courses. There was a very well stocked and ancient college library (this was before the days of computers and on-line databases) and we also had access to the main university library.

I could attend virtually any undergraduate or postgraduate lectures in the University. I briefly studied Greek and Roman philosophy and in more detail, the history of science. Classes within the college itself covered Old and New Testament studies, comparative religions and philosophy.

There were many extracurricular activities to choose from including music, tennis and social events with a 'theme'

- this was before the days of discotheques! I was introduced to croquet on the college lawn which, for the unfamiliar, is a sport that is said to be very character building because it is possible to be way ahead of the other players for most of a match and still loose to the player who until then has been last!

There was some interest from fellow students as to why I had decided to take this 'year out' and to be honest I quite enjoyed this curiosity. Most of the other postgradu-ates were from an arts or business background, and meeting a doctor as a colleague, rather than someone rather mystical only when you were unwell, must have been unusual for many of them. I made some good friends especially with those who could overcome the difficulty of thinking I was always seeing at them as potential patients!

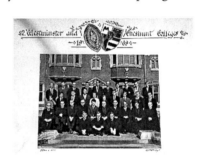

Some Personal Reflections
From My Time in Cambridge

Health and Love

- There are many ways to define 'health' and this varies in different cultures and religions, as well as through history. Understanding health requires the study of lin-guistics

- During the 19th century Industrial Revolution many scientists undertook the 'search for truth' from a deeply religious perspective
- Health can be seen as relating to the absence of disease or whether we see disease as normal, (most of us at all ages have a variety of illnesses) and our health relates to how we respond and adjust to this. It can be argued that most 'Health Services' are actually 'Disease Services' which is not to decry their importance, but recognizes that we can be both healthy and ill at the same time.
- The National 'Health Service' in the UK, founded in 1949, and has tended to encourage an unspoken belief that the state is fully responsible for our health. For example, the care for the elderly and the dying tend to become under-resourced since they are seen as a sign of failure.
- Health can be seen in the context of compassion, love and service 'in the moment' (e.g. as demonstrated in the parables of the Good Samaritan or the Prodigal Son) - not to be equated to sympathy or pity that can be experienced in front of the television.
- Health can also be seen as choosing 'God' (divine love) before 'Mammon' (variously translated as money or possessions) as our lifestyle guide. 'Mammon' is not condemned, it is simply a case of which comes first. A similar way of putting this is we can choose between 'the power of love' or 'the love of power'.
- 'Love' can be thought of as eros or agape. Eros being physical often self-centered love but not necessarily

the worse for this. Agape being love for all, friends and enemies, as we 'have been loved' or as we 'are loved'. Sadly, agape is often seen as solely a human experience and rarely includes love of our environment (all of creation).

- Spiritual love usually refers to love 'in the here and now' or to use a modern expression 'in the moment'. The term expresses many peoples experience that there is something around and yet seemingly beyond us that is truly worth pursuing - infinite love, the only human experience that outlives time and is everlasting. The Bible breathes of this experience particularly through the records we have of the life and teachings of the historical Jesus.

Science and Philosophy

- Science and philosophy both have a very similar definition that can be summarised as 'the search for truth using empirical (objective) observations with an attitude of disinterest and a sense of awe and wonder'.
- Science is a method of study and cannot decide for us what questions we should ask, (it can suggest ideas for further study) or how we should to use the knowledge gained.
- Titles and Words can mean different things to different people in different situations and at different periods of history. Basically, both verbal and textual communication has limitations. This requires intellectual modesty.
- We should respect statements from others but not accept

them at 'face value', employ understanding and modest criticism.

- The 'faults' we see in others often reflect our own uncertainties or mirror guilt about our own fantasies. 'Never laugh at others, just with them'.

- There is no such thing as 'absolute truth' or how to precisely distinguish 'good from evil' (e.g. the mathematical principle of uncertainty or the expulsion from the 'Garden of Eden' of Adam and Eve). Believing there is, either consciously or subconsciously, can lead at the best to misunderstandings and at the worst, catastrophes such as wars.

- Money can be a means to an end - but is not an end in itself.

Religion

- The biblical teachings progressively focus on an understanding of there being only one God with faith, hope and love being paramount. Eventually a total commitment to this belief, through the life and death of Jesus, clashes openly with self-centered, power and property seeking ambition which is a temptation for all of us and demonstrably transient.

- Religions may also focus on many gods, which may be represented through physical 'idols' although there are usually just one or two overall supreme deities. Less formalised beliefs include worship of ancestors and 'spiritual' experiences when it is sensed that there is something 'out there and beyond us, which profoundly influences our lives.

- When a religion is 'textually' based then understanding the writings requires availability of the texts and an ability to be able to read and interpret them. There can be a risk that an interpreter uses the texts to further personal opinions, power or ambitions particularly when directed towards the illiterate. These ambitions may be a quest for status or money.

- Texts can contain historical and reflective records, meaningful myths or inspirational writings written by a variety of authors. While much in terms of human behaviour and attitudes does not change, these writings benefit from being understood in the context of the times in which they were written.

- Individual records of the same event can differ, as would be expected, which can help increase our understanding of the spiritual messages, examples being two versions of creation and four versions of the resurrection in the Bible.

An Introduction to General Practice

During my sabbatical year, I undertook some general practice locums to help finance the course and accommodation costs.

In Cambridge

In Cambridge I helped out in a single handed practice and saw large numbers of student patients. I often felt somewhat out of my depth giving advice to students only a few years younger than myself about psychological problems and issues such as family planning. The oral contraceptive had only just become licensed and available and its role was still controversial.

In Haverfordwest in Wales

At the end of the sabbatical year I bought a second-hand Morris 1000 traveller estate car for £50 which was very reliable, and a big advantage was that most servicing and minor repairs could be managed myself with the help of a manual. There was plenty 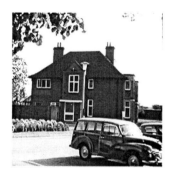 of room inside the engine compartment to move around and do jobs like servicing the carburettor and changing oil filters or spark plugs. I even was able to replace the clutch, fan and drive belts, brake cylinders, pipes and engine gaskets!

Having a car made it possible for me to go Haverford-west in South Wales, where I worked for a month with two brothers who had inherited the practice from their father. They had turned down the option of moving into a new health centre in the town, remaining instead in the home of one of the doctors. It was a very traditional family practice. A very attentive live-in housekeeper looked after me. One of the brothers took me up in his private mini-plane and the engine bonnet blew open after take off making it difficult to see where we were going! He blamed the co-owner for not fastening it down correctly. After landing and sorting out the problem we had an interesting flight that included flying underneath a bridge over the Cleddau River. I doubt if this was normally allowed but he was a local doctor and in those days local doctors tended to get away with a lot of things: including being let off car speeding tickets!

The experience was overall very relaxed, before the days of computers, continual form filling and relatively few medications were available. My father had told me that 'GP' stood for 'grateful patients' and on the whole I think this is still the case. It was possible to go for a swim in the sea between house visits.

I was very new to general practice and as mentioned previously we had no training at medical school in those days in many, probably most, of the common illnesses seen outside hospitals. One day I saw a number of rashes in children that I thought might be allergies until a very pleasant grandmother said to me, "Do you think it might be german measles, doctor?" I had to go back to the patients I had seen earlier and explain my mistake!

I regularly visited an army caravan site where many young wives were living with young children on their own. Their husbands were away and they had no family support. One mother was very distressed because her newborn baby had had diarrhoea for 3 days. She was in tears, had already been up to the surgery and had a previous house visit. I decided that a short admission would be appropriate in these circumstances, but later received a 'shirty' discharge letter from the junior hospital doctor saying it was an inappropriate admission because the child was not seriously dehydrated. This made me very aware of how medical training at that time, based only in hospitals, largely ignored the fact that social circumstances can make managing illness at home very difficult and potentially dangerous.

One other interesting experience was prescribing a 'tonic' for a patient who was a bit 'run down'. I found one in the British National Formulary of that time called 'tinc. stryc'. In my innocence I had no idea this contained strychnine in a very homeopathic dose. The patient read the prescription and fortunately, being an elderly man with a gentle manner, did not immediately imagine I was trying to poison him. However, he came back to get reassurance from one of the other doctors who prescribed something containing vitamin C as an alternative! I don't think strychnine is now in the formulary.

POSTGRADUATE YEARS TRAINING AS A GENERAL PHYSICIAN

Obstetrics

I enjoyed the experience I gained during this 9-month post where patients normally go away with something rather than with something removed! I had responsibility in outpatients and on post-natal wards as well as in the labour suite. After a few months I became proficient in most procedures including assisted deliveries (although not quite the same as the methods I had used to delivered calves on the farm with a piece of rope and lots of strength!). I was confident with episiotomies, epidurals and removing retained placentae and I suspect many of these roles are now only performed by more experienced doctors. We went out regularly as members of the 'flying squad' to homes where something was going wrong with home deliveries. At this time there was a move towards all deliveries being in hospital, which is very understandable. However, many mothers, especially those who already had a number of children, did not like this and preferred to be at home. When my mother had her children, going to hospital for delivery was only when there were complications. Now, with most deliveries being in hospital, maternal and infant death rates have fallen to very low levels in the UK, in contrast to countries without these facilities freely available. There seems now to be a partial move back to home deliveries, which mothers are free to choose. These deliveries are supervised by very experienced midwives, and normally take place after modern scanning and other investigations make complications unlikely.

Something that is not likely to happen now in the UK, is the very distressing situation where babies are born with multiple or serious abnormalities that had not been recognised during pregnancy. Ultrasound scans and diagnostic blood tests were not available. I remember when a mother I had been looking after delivered her baby with anencephaly, a rapidly lethal condition. You can imagine how difficult it was to explain this to her after she had delivered when she had been very excited at the prospect of having a healthy baby. My obstetric experience came in very useful later when working in Indian villages.

Infectious and Tropical Diseases

This senior house officer post at East Birmingham Hospital where I had worked previously was my introduction to these specialities, which were to be the focus of my interests for most of the rest of my career. At that time it involved the care of both children and adults. However, children's hospitals now normally have their own isolation units and the highly contagious and potentially lethal diseases such as diphtheria and scarlet fever are no longer major threats.

We saw a wide range of diarrhoeal illnesses, pneumonia, jaundice, meningitis, glandular fever, shingles, unexplained fevers, unusual rashes and illnesses contracted abroad. One of the consultants had previously been a professor in Sudan. I became quickly aware of how little training in these sorts of problems had been covered at medical school. Now the major problems are resistant bacteria, norovirus (the cause of what was previously only known as winter vomiting disease), HIV and hepatitis infections and hospital acquired infections such as C. difficile.

We saw many very contagious, normally childhood, infections such as measles, mumps, whooping cough and chickenpox (we used to say this virus could crawl around the floor between cubicles) for which there are vaccines.

The pattern of infections in the UK has changed dramatically over the last 100 years. For example, my aunt

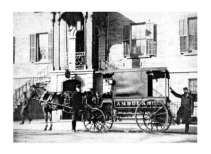

could describe very clearly how in the 1910s she was admitted to an isolation hospital in Scotland in a horse-drawn ambulance with a friend from school. They both had diphtheria from which she recovered, but her friend did not. Ruchill Infectious Diseases Hospital in Glasgow where I worked after my return from India had been the ambulance centre for the north of Glasgow and still had its stables used then as store houses.

I also visited one of my uncle's in the 1950s in a tuberculosis sanatorium where he was being looked after. This was when rest, fresh air and good diet were seen as the cornerstones of tuberculosis treatment and drug treatment was not yet established. When I went to India, it was in many ways like going back to seeing the disease patterns of

Victorian times and the early 20th century.

Broad general medical knowledge was necessary because many illnesses seen were not due to infection such as inflammatory bowel disease, cholangitis causing jaundice and tumours causing cerebral or pulmonary symptoms - all of which were initially thought to have been due to infection.

With my previous student experience in Africa, I was especially interested in infections that had been contracted abroad such as malaria, typhoid, tuberculosis, leprosy, intestinal helminths and amoebic hepatitis. I remember admitting a slaughter man with cutaneous anthrax who had never been out of the UK. He had been scratching his eyebrow after dismembering a cow. 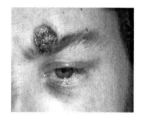 I recognised it immediately because of my time spent in Africa where this disease was common - these days in the UK this would have been a national news item!

Towards the end of this post, one of the infectious diseases consultants, Dr Alisdair Geddes, suggested to me that it would be valuable to spend some time in clinical pathology as a sound basis for a future infectious or tropical disease career. I accepted this advice and my training involved haematology, including examining blood films and bone marrow aspirations, microbiology, histology and undertaking postmortems on a daily basis. At that time, the relatives of any patient who died were asked for permission to perform a post-mortem examination. Now, with much more effective non-invasive investigation procedures being available, such as body scans, postmortems are no longer routinely necessary to determine a cause of death.

General Medicine

After finishing my time at East Birmingham Hospital, I decided to complete my training as a general physician and study for membership of the Royal College of Physicians. I had been turned down by the 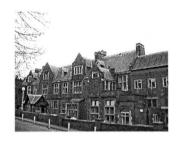 teaching hospital where I did my junior medical house job for their full-time resident medical officer post. I was by then married with one son and the post involved permanently 'living-in' the hospital for one year which I was not prepared to undertake. However, I then found a registrar post in St Cross Hospital Rugby (above) where there were two medical consultants. One was younger, up-to-date and enthusiastic; the other elderly, greatly respected by his patients, but with serious chronic health problems including alcoholism and this meant I had to take on a lot of responsibility for his patients. While this was not ideal, and probably would not be acceptable now, I gained a lot of personal experience in decision-making and always had the other consultant to call on if needed.

Saint Cross was 15 miles away from the facilities of a big city hospital, and it was more like a large community 'cottage hospital' where staff all knew each other and local general practitioners would regularly come in to see how their patients were getting on. I often met previous patients when going shopping in the town.

There was no junior house officer to help but the admission rate was usually about five patients each day so the workload was manageable. There was one male and one female ward of the Nightingale type with 15 patient beds in each and two single rooms for seriously ill patients. We had one electrocardiogram (ECG) machine, which was used by the whole hospital. There was one cardiac monitor and a postoperative but no high dependency rooms. Our outpatient department was small and three of us carried out consultations around a large table with little privacy but we had curtained off cubicles for examinations. This may now seem rather primitive but it all seemed to work well with credit due to the sensitivity and thoughtfulness of the nursing and auxiliary staff. This set-up was also good experience for working in India later on. While being responsible full-time for the ward during the day, there was cover on alternate nights and weekends by staff from the paediatric and chest units.

I became good friends with an Indian gynaecology registrar who got into trouble for bringing his surgical waiting list down too much by working late in evenings with the support of the theatre staff. The problem was that efficiency led to a reduction in the resources provided by the health board! Another medical colleague was from Pakistan, and it was he who suggested I wrote to the Vellore Christian

Medical College in India to enquire about work there (as described in the following chapter). An amusing aside was that when we had him round for an evening meal, I offered him some homemade elderflower 'champagne'. He enjoyed it but became very 'chatty' and I had wrongly thought it was non-alcoholic. He was a Muslim for whom drinking alcohol is taboo. I should have known since the process involved the production of bubbles of carbon dioxide as the result of fermentation so there must have been a few drops of alcohol in it - but we remained good friends!

Our accommodation was in a flat in what used to be the Rugby workhouse. It was half a mile from the medical wards, and to travel across involved a pleasant walk or cycle across a park. The rest of this building was derelict and I used the empty room above the flat to grow mushrooms; until water began to creep though the flat's ceiling! There was an area of garden, originally part of the workhouse, where I grew vegetables and was very upset when a beautiful cauliflower, which I had nurtured from seed, was stolen. I reported it to the police but they just laughed!

Because there were no other medical wards the experience I gained was immense and covered all specialities. We had weekly clinical meetings attended by both hospital doctors and the general practitioners that allowed discussions over co-ordinated patient care. On Sunday mornings, once a month, a Professor Arnott from Birmingham came over to join in a case review meeting. I had known him from medical student days and he was a family friend as well, having trained at Edinburgh at the same time as my father.

He was a chief examiner for the London Royal Medical College of Physicians and this helped me a lot in my preparation for the membership (MRCP) examination. He was even there to 'say hullo' when I went down to London for the clinical part of the exam, which was reassuring. I hope he did not influence the examiners!

It was a happy time in Rugby, although hard work and an example of 'small is beautiful' in terms of lifestyle and links with the local community; involvement not so easily experienced in big hospitals in cities.

At around this time my father retired and my parents moved house with my sister to Shrawley, 'The Knapp' in a village in another part of Worcestershire. It was in an attractive area but very different from the close community I had enjoyed around Hollow Tree House. I believe the move was partly to facilitate my sister's interest in riding because the new house had several acres of land attached. It was clear my parents missed their friends around Bromsgrove and in Tardebigge; I visited during weekends and holidays.

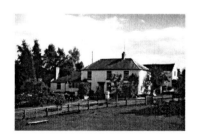

INDIAN EXPERIENCE
IN RURAL HEALTH CARE

Why India?

My interest in working abroad at some stage after completing my UK postgraduate training was sparked by my time in Zimbabwe as a medical student. I had also worked on an infectious diseases unit where we regularly saw patients who had contracted illnesses abroad. When working as a medical registrar in Rugby, I became friendly with a doctor from Pakistan who said, 'Why not write to the Christian Medical College Hospital (CMCH) in Vellore?' This internationally renowned institution, was staffed predominantly by Indian nationals, but welcomed doctors from abroad with expertise that fitted their needs. I received a reply (before the days of emails) inviting me to join one of their medical units. The post I was offered was as a lecturer in medicine which at that time was validated by Madras University. Later CMCH gained independent medical school status.

Preparation

UK sponsorship was necessary since non-Indians could not be paid a salary in India and I was accepted by the Council for World Mission (CWM), an inter-denomination organisation that already had Indian links. Initially the personnel officer at CWM encouraged me to consider working in a small village in Papua New Guinea because CMCH already had sufficient medical staff, but it was very remote and the only realistic way to travel there was by sea. I felt it was more of a role for an experienced general practitioner and travelling with two young children to an area with a mortality rate for the under 5 year olds approaching 50%, seemed to be taking an inappropriate risk. It was required that we spent 3 months preparation at Selly Oak Colleges in Birmingham studying anthropology, culture and teaching methods. I felt at the time this was a bit excessive, and learning on the spot would have been preferable. However, it was a useful period and allowed time to obtain the necessary Indian visas.

While at Selly Oak I was introduced, by a theological professor from Bangalore, to the 'arrows or circles' concept that has been used to describe culture as in the West as focusing on 'ambition and wealth' in contrast to Hindu culture focusing on 'relationships'. He considered the former approach to be more consistent with Judeo-Greek than Christian teaching. After some time in India, I came to understand what he meant as demonstrated through traditional Indian family loyalties and village cohesion. This is all the more important when there is no government welfare system or means of 'buying' your way out of difficulties. The 'wealth come first' approach has taken hold in many countries such as the UK where consumerism seems to have taken over as society's norm in the vain hope that money can buy you health and happiness. 'You cannot worship God and Mammon (money)' - Luke 6:23. This is not to the exclusion of one or the other but one has to take priority.

I was already very interested in environmental and

ecological issues which got me into trouble at the College. I kept turning off the heating in the very large clothes drying room when there was nothing hanging up to dry. I also tried, without success, to convince the gardener that walking on the lawn might be allowed, at least at weekends!

Eventually we set off in 1973 on one of the first Jumbo-Jets for the 15-hour journey via Bombay (now Mumbai) with our 3 year old and 6 month old sons. In Madras, later renamed Chennai after the village where British traders first built a settlement, the airport arrivals lounge was a building made of bamboo, boarding and thatch. Since then, I have flown well over 20 times to and from India, and watched the airport grow progressively into a modern international hub.

The Christian Medical College and Hospital (CMCH) Vellore

This institution was founded early in the 20th century as a medical school for female doctors. Its founding was inspired by Dr Ida Scudder, the daughter of an American missionary, who recognised that women were dying in childbirth because they would not accept care from male doctors. It is now internationally recognised as a centre of excellent medical care that aims to run the delicate balance between providing high modern standards of care with low cost effective care for those who cannot afford, or do not wish, the allopathic ('Western') approach.

On arrival we were disappointed to be given accommodation in a small upstairs flat on the very crowded campus of the main hospital in the centre of the town. This was not what we had hoped for coming from a rural background. However, something very striking from the start was the friendliness of neighbours and others as well as a genuine understanding of the stresses we were experiencing - now called 'culture shock'. In the absence of radio and television, it was very normal practice to regularly visit neighbours, share meals and make your own entertainment with discussions, singing, storytelling and playing games of all sorts. Young children were welcomed at evening activities and if they fell asleep you just carried them home to bed - there was no obsession with strict bedtimes. For many of us 'cat napping' during the day was an art well worth practicing especially around midday during the hot season.

Our time in Selly Oak Colleges had not prepared us for our arrival into serious and repeated union strikes that had been going on in the hospital for several years, made all the more stressful because we had two young children. All gates into the campus had been barred up or walled over, except for one that was staffed by security guards. Signs saying, 'Go home foreigners' were on display, and on occasion staff were advised not to leave the hospital, and slept in their offices. These strikes had a political dimension which was said to be linked to a wish by the regional state government to take over the running of the hospital. We had been allocated a cook and housekeeper whose husband turned out to be one of the strike leaders. However, she was very supportive, stayed with us throughout our time at CMCH, and even went with us during the summers to one of the hill stations, which was normal practice for expatriates unused to the extreme heat.

I initially had a feeling of self-consciousness being one of very few with white skin which made you immediately recognisable as probably someone linked to the previous imperial power. I had little knowledge of Tamil, but I quickly learned that much could be conveyed through gestures and other forms of body language. 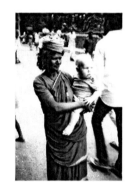 Also, English is the second language taught in schools in South India, unlike in the north where it is Hindi.

In general, very little animosity was however shown towards foreigners; indeed the opposite was the case. However, on more than one occasion, when crossing the picket lines outside the hospital, the police had to usher me to safety, away from the threat of having the contents of bedpans, or worse, thrown at me.

Our stay in the hospital was for only a few months, after which I was moved as a locum physician in the Leprosy Research Centre, which was in a rural area just outside the town. This was a relief, especially when we felt safety was an issue with our children. The Hospital's medical director arranged this despite his heavy involvement in managing the strikes. This was an example of the hospital's policy caring for its individual staff and not confining itself to financial, business and strategic plans, which now seem to be the focus of much of the administration in the UK's health service. While both relationships and money are important in our modern world, we have to choose which of these should be our priority.

Eventually the national government intervened in the unrest, which was being replicated in other parts of the country, and declared a national state of emergency. The local state governor was removed and strikes were temporarily banned. We even had a morale-boosting visit by helicopter from Mrs Ghandi, the Indian Prime Minister at the time.

Secondment to Karigiri Leprosy Research Centre

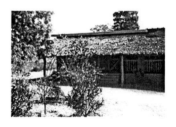

This lasted about 6 months and I gained a very valuable insight into the issues involved in the diagnosis, treatment and care of patients with leprosy. Karigiri had charitable status and therefore unions were not allowed. Consequently there were no strikes, despite it being associated with CMCH. The relaxed atmosphere allowed me to be more focused on, and in control of, my professional tasks. Our accommodation (above) was very rural, with all that goes with this: snakes, scorpions, water shortages and frequent electricity cuts. However, none of these things caused serious difficulties, and we learned from other staff how to be prepared with water tubs and candles. One of the rules was that snakes were to be treated with respect and not killed except in exceptional circumstances. Snakes are not naturally aggressive unless they are seeking prey, so they rarely attack humans except when accidentally stood on or attacked.

Karigiri was famous for the pioneering work of Dr Paul Brand, an American by birth, who developed pioneering techniques including tendon sheath incision and transplants for those with impending sensory or established motor nerve damage due to leprosy. Along with our work in the hospital, we held village clinics in surrounding districts to identify new cases, provide follow-up and supply medications to those who could not, or would not, travel to the Centre. Since the advent of the bactericidal drug rifampicin 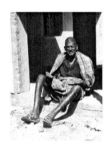 (kills the organisms, rapidly reducing the spread of infection) new cases of leprosy have become rare in much of India. This patient has the lepromatous form which has caused anesthesia of his hands and feet with resulting digit loss due to repeated injuries.

It is spread mainly through organisms in infected nasal secretions, so regular close contact and poor hygiene are important factors, encouraging its spread in conditions of cramped housing. In the absence of handkerchiefs, 'blowing your nose' usually involved putting a finger or thumb over one nostril and snorting out the phlegm - an excellent means of transmission!

The Rural Health Centre

After leaving Karigiri, I joined CMCH's Rural Health Centre based near its College campus. The campus is 5km outside the Vellore town and I was happy to be able to continue 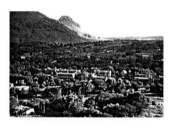 working in a rural environment. It is also where most of the pre-clinical teaching takes place, and many staff and all students live.

I was given responsibilities for serving nine villages, which involved daily clinics held in small public buildings such as temple entrances or villager's houses. I worked with public health nurses who spoke both Tamil and English. A big difference from the UK was that primary clinical care, preventive medicine and public health were effectively one speciality, so there was no split between seeing sick patients and working out how various ailments could have been prevented.

We undertook regular evening educational activities in the villages with use of flip charts, play-acting and games, and regularly involved the junior doctors and students.

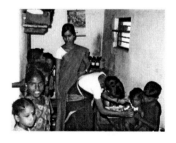 Junior doctors helped me undertake simple epidemiological studies, for example, when a village was found to have a particular local health issue such as filariasis, leprosy, scabies, hookworm or cholera.

The findings of these simple studies were then used to set up appropriate preventive measures. The majority of medical students studying at CMCH were from urban backgrounds and we started annual 'community orientation programmes' for them, that involved living in a village for a week to build up close relationships with selected families. The students undertook simple demographic studies and kept in touch with these families throughout their whole five year course. A different village was visited each year, and this programme, started while I was there in the 1970s, is still ongoing today.

Working at the Rural Health Centre, I became familiar with the daily activities of farmers: the crops they grew, the care of the animals, such as cows, buffalo, sheep, goats, ducks and chickens. Activities revolved around the seasons where winter was cooler following the major monsoon in November and summer was very hot especially during April to July. Most cultivation and harvesting took place in the winter months when straw and hay for animal feed was stored for use during the hot, dry summers - the opposite way around to farming life in the UK. There were never frosts and being close to the equator, the duration of day and night was fairly equal which allowed most crops to grow throughout the year dependent, of course, on adequate rainfall.

Village Life

The sort of things that were sometimes unfamiliar to students brought up in urban areas included farming practices, but also the wide variety of locally-sourced house building materials. Bamboo and palm leaf used to thatch roofs, and mud mixed with cow dung to plaster walls, giving protection against erosion in the rain. Walls and roofs were sometimes made from tiles using local clay. Very few houses had indoor toilets: the fields and roadside were used instead. Flush toilets are not possible when water is scare. In any case, toileting inside the house is often considered disgusting and dirty, as it was in many countries, including Britain, before the days of water closets. Personal washing and bathing was usually undertaken outside behind a simple screen using water in small quantities poured over the body with cups. In contrast to cities, begging was rare within villages where the local community normally took care of widows and the destitute. The main village was usually separate from the 'Harijan' (previously 'outcastes') area, although there was no obvious antagonism between the different castes. While accepting things are changing, at this time, telephones, electric lights and electronic equipment such as televisions were very unusual.

Often, established practices are developed over generations with good reason, although the science behind these practices may not have been obvious at the time. One example of this is the normal practice in India of boiling milk before it is consumed, which suggests that a link

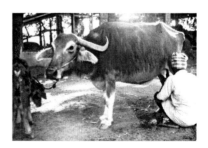

between diseases such as tuberculosis and unpasturised milk may have been recognised many generations ago. Another example was the use of a roadside plant called phyllanthus amarus, which was boiled and given to those with jaundice. This observation introduced me to scientific colleagues in Chennai, and led to a continuing collaboration after my return to the UK as discussed later. In my experience most people throughout the world are very pragmatic, and if a new medical treatment for a disease is seen to be effective, it is quickly accepted.

It was clear there was a real need for low cost effective care, and a preventive medicine approach. I attempted to write a village healthcare manual, which focused on cheap and easily available remedies.

Cooking was mostly carried out using kerosene (or bottled gas) stoves. Those who could not afford this, used either wood, or a mixture of cow dung and straw made into cakes and dried in the sun. Using wood for fuel has led to major environmental problems whereby trees are destroyed and not replaced. This situation is an interesting contrast to Britain where wood is seen as a renewable source of heating. I was not aware of a Tamil word for 'rubbish' since most waste was recycled in one way or another. As in other countries however, plastic bags have more recently been causing a major problem.

Farming

With my rural and farming background, I felt privileged to

have been able to follow the whole yearly cycle of Indian village life: caring for the soil, planting, harvesting, animal husbandry and the, all-important, monsoon rains.

The whole village community was involved in local food production. For example, the men undertook activities involving cattle such as ploughing, transporting products to market and drawing water from wells. Women were respon- sible for planting and 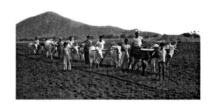 harvesting rice. After the monsoon rains, it was common for the schools to close allowing children to help with planting and harvesting of groundnuts. This allowed the whole process to be done quickly to take advantage of the soil while it was wet. This is an interesting comparison with Scotland, where children were given time off to go 'tattie howking' (potato picking).

Water management is a vital part of the rural life, especially where monsoons are not always sufficient to provide water for a full year. Shortages after failed monsoons can quickly lead to famine and malnutrition; requiring feeding programmes with food being brought in from elsewhere in the country. I witnessed 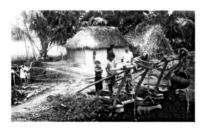 this first hand after three years of failed monsoons. This picture shows the traditional means of raising water out of an agricultural well using a cow to raise the water, a rope and a large leather bladder. Water tankers were a common sight especially in the cities.

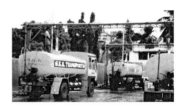

Monoculture (just one crop on a plot of land) was used for certain water hungry crops such as rice, ragi (the 'poor man's' cereal which makes delicious porridge) as well as bananas and sugar cane. Polyculture was used for growing vegetables such as pulses, aubergines, beans and pumpkins. Carrots, potatoes and other temperate climate vegetables, as well as grapes, apples and oranges were imported daily by train or lorry from cooler climes in the hills. Some tree seedpods were used as vegetables or for flavouring such as the 'drumstick' and the tamarind. Popular fruits included the banana, mango, guava, custard apple and papaya.

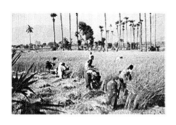

Mangos are seasonal and very valuable so all day and night 'guards' are often employed to protect them when they are close to harvesting. The variety and presentation of fruit and vegetables in Vellore market was fascinating for foreigners but also, in my experience, for locals who enjoy spending time wandering around and indulging in some good humoured bargaining.

Village animals included cattle, water buffalo, goats, sheep, ducks and chickens. Wild creatures include the mongoose, rats (including the giant bandicoot), frogs, (whose the croaking in the evenings after rains is legendary), many stray dogs and the occasional jackal.

It was clear to me that the 'sacred cow' expression is a misconception, probably invented by the British who did not live close enough to the villagers to appreciate how important the cow's role is in village life. The cow is certainly revered, but not worshiped in the sense that many religions use this word, because it has a vital role. I like to see the cow's role as comparable to motorcars upon which so many of us are utterly dependent for our day-to-day activities - our 'sacred' motorcars!

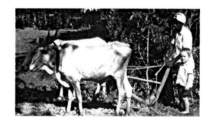

There was a huge variety of birds and butterflies, as well as adders, cobras, vipers, scorpions (always good to look inside your shoes before you put them on) and white ants which are termites that eat dead wood and create large mounds of soil as nests. Bees are active throughout the year, unlike in countries with cold winters, and their combs are often visible in trees or under archways of buildings and temples. Less popular are the mosquitoes!

Observations on Health Issues in the Villages During the 1970s: Mothers, Infants and Child Care

After marriage the bride normally goes to stay with the husband's family but when she becomes pregnant, and delivery approaches, she returns to her mother's home. In the village situation, the women continue their normal household activities and work, such as planting and harvesting crops such as rice or 'paddy', right up until she is ready to give birth. If the daughter does not live in the grandmother's village, she may have to travel to her mother's house in advance.

If a woman is thought to be infertile then she should go out at night without being seen, and hang a cow's placenta in a banyan tree wrapped in a cloth. The banyan tree with its many hanging root stems is a symbol of fertility.

Traditionally, local village midwives (dais) conduct deliveries, and these skills are passed on from mother to daughter. There is little, if any, antenatal care and it is not uncommon, for example, for women during pregnancy to be very anaemic, often due to chronic hookworm infection from working in the paddy fields.

Within the area now served by the CMCH Rural Health Centre, the dais are trained in the basics of antenatal care. Mothers are also seen, if necessary, by training nursing and medical staff in the Health Centre, where the majority of deliveries are now conducted. This is a big change in practice and much safer. There has been little resistance to this move from the dais, whose status has been increased by training in antenatal care and in basic first aid. CMC pioneered this adjustment of responsibilities, which is now followed in many parts of the world. Major improvements

include, for example, a reduction in unrecognized pre-ec-
lampsia, serious perineal tears during delivery and deaths
due to gross bleeding and retained placentae. Prior to these
changes, death as a result of pregnancy was very common,
just as it was in Britain 200 years ago. However, there
remains a huge difference in standards of care in many parts
of the country, especially between urban and rural settings
where effective care during severe illness or complications
may be many hours away from the mother's home village.
The 'ambulance' would usually be a bullock cart, bicycle or
possibly a rickshaw.

Some Further Medical Observations

A common entry point for neonatal tetanus infection is
the umbilical cord, which may be cut with unsterile blades
and then covered with dry cow dung for 'protection'. Otitis
media, or middle ear infection, where the eardrum has
ruptured can also allow tetanus spore to flourish.

In the areas I worked in, measles was commonly
believed to be caused by a visitation from the Goddess
Mariamma and so management was designed to please her.
This includes keeping the child in a dark room and restricting
fluids. The death rate was around 40%. The reason for these
practices related to reducing the photophobia since bright
lights make it more uncomfortable and restricting fluid was
seen to be a way to control diarrhoea since it seemed logical
that the drinks just 'go straight through and out the other
end'.

'Dhosham' was the local term used for severe dehydration that was taken as a sign that the child is almost certain to die. On one occasion we sat giving small amounts of fluid orally to such a child for a few hours despite the concern of the mother that this was wrong. However, the child was running 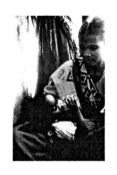 around the next day and this event convinced many villagers that some of our allopathic medicine and ways of treatment could be trusted.

Congenital and rheumatic heart disease was common and normally meant early death since surgery was either unavailable, too expensive or the parents found the idea of surgery unacceptable. It is often said that rheumatic heart disease declined in the UK because of a change in the organism's virulence - my impression was that this decline was more likely due to the widespread use of antibiotics in more serious throat and skin infections, since it is now much rarer in India too.

Lobar pneumonia was common in both children and young adults and antibiotic treatment was often delayed or not considered. Untreated, the death rate was around 10% and this was the experience in the UK before antibiotics were available as well.

Chickenpox was common in young adults but less common in young children. This may because children rarely wandered outside their villages and local schools, which may reduce the likelihood of outbreaks.

The very few toilets tended to be dry, very dirty and rarely cleaned out. This meant the fields and public ground like the verges of roads and railway lines were used and in town, the roadside. This practice provided the ideal setting for the spread of typhoid, cholera, giardiasis and amoebiasis and other gastrointestinal infections.

Tuberculosis was, and still is, extremely common and frequently found to be present together with other conditions.

Leprosy was common and interestingly, discrimination rare. Sufferers lived normal lives in the villages. Only if they had no family support and became so crippled they could not work, did they take up begging to make an income.

I had heard previously in the UK, that diabetes was very rare in both India and Africa - this was clearly incorrect. Maybe this applied previously for type 2 diabetes related to diet and it is likely that those with type 1 diabetes rapidly resulted in death in the hot climate when no insulin was available. Even the government hospitals had times when they had no insulin available, and it is easy to understand the difficulties of giving daily injections in the village situation.

Suicide is often related to family feuds or poverty, and hanging was the usual means for men and poisoning or drowning in a well for women. The seeds of certain trees are known to be very poisonous - one such tree used to grow outside the Rural Health Centre but it has now been removed.

Herbal remedies were available for many conditions such as fever and respiratory infections.

Tooth caries were rare due to little use of food and drink containing refined sugar but gingivitis is very common. Teeth cleaning was done with wood ash and toothpicks.

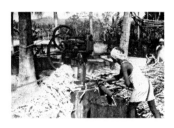

The local practice for fractured limbs was to be wrapped in bandages containing leaves from the Neem tree - manipulation was at times refused when offered. Injuries were common especially when machinery was used without effective safety procedures in place, for example when of crushing sugarcane to extract the juice (above).

Chewing beetle nut can lead to red staining and mouth cancer, and the nuts are usually wrapped in tobacco leaves.

Travelling in India

On the roads

It is said that Indians are among the world's greatest travellers and this certainly appears likely considering the volume of people using the roads. It is not just motorised vehicles, but pedestrians, cyclists and bullock carts. An enormous change

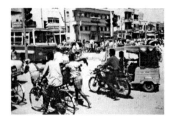

since the 1970s is the volume of traffic which, as in many other cities around the world, seems to now be constantly gridlocked during the daytime. Road accidents are a major problem both in the cities and especially on faster main trunk roads because of traffic congestion. On rural roads the speed is much faster, therefore serious accidents and fatalities are common. Traffic coming in opposite directions tend to play 'cat and mouse' to see who will get out of the way first, which is especially scary when there is only a single

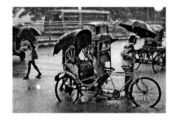

tarmacadamed lane. Experienced passengers often prefer to sit in the back seat and go to sleep or pray! I have witnessed many cars, lorries, buses and rickshaws seriously damaged, overturned or smashed. Maintenance of vehicles is also a problem. Travel during monsoons also causes problems.

I tend to wheeze during hay fever seasons but also when traffic fumes are bad and there is little wind to circulate the air. I have experienced this mildly in many places including Glasgow, but the only very bad asthma attack I have had was in Calcutta (now Kolkata) due to diesel fumes from lorries, buses, taxis and rickshaws. My escape was to enter the underground for a rest and to recover - the trains used electricity.

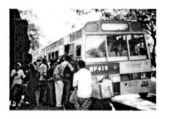

Air Travel

I tend to be an anxious traveller, not because of fear of flying, but because of all the uncertainties that travel can bring. This is perhaps surprising when I had been able to go off as a teenager with a friend, a rucksack and £100 to explore Europe, with no plans as to where we would go or what we would do. This must be something to do with lack of awareness at a young age of all the challenges that might lie ahead.

Once I forgot my passport, which I only discovered after arriving by shuttle plane in London, so I had to change my flight and go back to Glasgow to collect it. At this time, phone calls to and within India were unreliable so I had difficultly letting my hosts in Chennai know what had happened. Consequently I was not met in the airport and had to find emergency accommodation in a nearby hotel while things were sorted out. On another trip when I had been having a particularly stressful time in the city on my own, I went to the airport with a good book and stayed for a couple of hours reading in the restaurant before returning to the tasks in hand. I find there is a sort of security feeling in airports despite the crowds and anonymity.

I have experienced two aborted landings, once when there was a cow on the runway in Bombay (now Mumbai) and once when returning to Heathrow. The pilot's light confirming the landing wheels were in place, did not light up, so the plane had to undertake a trial landing so visual check could be made by ground staff. Our eventual landing was accompanied by a string of fire engines and ambulances.

An amusing experience was on one occasion, after landing in Chennai we were unable to disembark for several hours because the plane had parked next to a truck. This made it impossible to open the aircraft doors. The driver of the truck had gone home with the keys!

I got myself particularly stressed when flying out to India at the time when Russia had just invaded Afghanistan. This was during the Cold War and there was a lot of talk about world conflict and the use of nuclear weapons. Partly, I think because I had just taken chloroquine for malaria prevention on an empty stomach, I was violently sick in Heathrow airport and ended up in their medical centre. I was checked over, given an anti-emetic, and after much pressing of buttons, was taken by wheelchair to the plane before anyone else, given three seats all to myself, tucked in and had a wonderful nights sleep!

Train Journeys

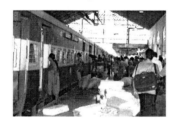 Train journeys in India are an experience few unfamiliar will forget. Like in the UK most train journeys are taken for long distance journeys or for commuting into cities for work. However many long distance journeys are overnight and there is a very efficient reserved seat system where you can book to travel in a variety of carriage types: air-conditioned aircraft seat type coaches, simple wooden benches or cabins with pull down bunk beds. The cheaper unbooked carriages can be very crowded but there are ticket inspectors who check up on whether passengers in reserved carriages have booked and are in the correct seat.

For those who are unfamiliar with train travel, fellow passengers are often very helpful when advice is needed. Local travellers are normally very ready to help foreigners and even share snacks and

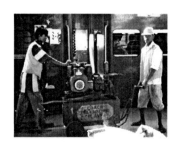

drinks. Toilets are very variable in type and cleanliness; this photo is of a toilet cleaning apparatus

The experience starts in the stations where it can be challenging to be sure you get into the correct carriage since the trains are often extremely long. There are however always porters to help you find your seat and carry your luggage - some stations have fixed porter charges but you will rarely get away without paying a generous tip.

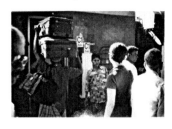

Train journeys are an opportunity for tourists who normally only visit the cities to see something of the country-side, crops such as rice, sugar cane, palm trees, papaya etc.
and cows, water buffalo and goats in their rural surroundings. Overnight travellers are usually interested to see that the sides of railways tracks are used in the early morning as toilets.

Holidays in the hill stations
Many of those who could afford it, which included most of the expatriates, would travel for a few weeks at the height

of the summer to a hill station for relief from the heat. The heat in the middle of the day was such that I found cycling slowly was much more pleasant than walking. In the main hospital, for logistical reasons, working throughout the day was usual, and it was difficult to be able to take a midday siesta.

Kodaikanal is one of two hill stations in Tamil Nadu. The road up was steep and long with many bends, and the possibility of the bus tumbling back down to the plains below seemed very real. The small town had a relaxed holiday atmosphere and there were many walks along the hillsides with views down onto the flat plains below. We stayed in a simple cottage and occasionally had a fire at night to keep warm and to heat water for bathing in a tin bath in the kitchen. Many of the plants and flowers were similar to those seen in the UK, most likely because they had been brought out by generations of expatriates before us as cuttings or seeds. Lettuce and strawberries were particularly welcome since they could not grow in the heat of the plains below.

There was a lake where we could hire rowing boats and on one occasion while rowing close to another boat, the male passenger and I started looking at each other with a sense of recognition. When we plucked up the courage to introduce ourselves, it turned out we had been to Bromsgrove school together - not close friends but there was enough in our memories to realise we had met before!

The other hill station was Ootacamund and there was a mountain railway as an alternative way of ascending.

These hills were more spread out and the ground was very fertile. It was from here that temperate fruits such as apples and oranges and vegetables including potatoes and carrots were grown and then exported down to the cities below by lorry or train. Horse riding was one of the enjoyable pastimes and it 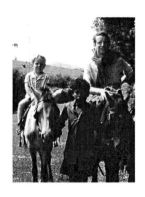 is said that snooker and billiards were invented here in the 'Englishman's club'.

A Holiday in Kashmir: Train, Plane and Sledging

The journey involved a two-day train trip from Chennai to Delhi with our children in a carriage that had a compartment with sleeping bunks. Somehow, the journey went fairly peacefully although the biggest problem was the less than pleasant toilet facilities. We made regular stops at stations where noise levels increased while passengers embarked and disembarked and food and drink sellers briefly invaded the train to sell their wares. We stopped en route in Agra to see around the Taj Mahal, which was much smaller than we expected.

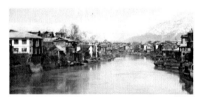 Before leaving Vellore, we had to obtain cholera vaccination certificates. The vaccine was administered in a government vaccination centre in the town where the needles were

reused, they were sharpened on a matchbox and sterilised in the flame of a candle. This was only in the early days of concerns about blood borne infections but was also a cost saving exercise.

In Kashmir we had to undergo more immigration security than when entering other Indian airports because of its disputed territory status. However, we were not aware at that time of any major threat to our safety and the, mostly Moslem, population were very friendly. It was winter, so the change from the heat of South India to snow and freezing conditions was quite dramatic. However, we were prepared in terms of clothing and the houseboat we stayed in had a wood stove.

We stayed on a barge and during the first afternoon we lost our 5-year-old son and we had thoughts of his body being carried down the Jhelum River to Pakistan: before we found him after 5-10 minutes underneath the very thick bed duvet. On a lighter note, we went on a bus trip up a nearby mountain to enjoy the snow but found that there was no bus back until the next day! We returned by toboggan, which did not take long because the toboggan driver went vertically down the mountain avoiding all the hairpins by crossing the road repeatedly at speed - fortunately there was no traffic coming!

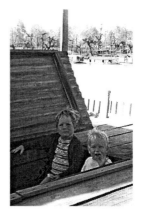

GENERAL PRACTICE
AFTER RETURN FROM INDIA

Although the time spent living in India was relatively brief, returning to the UK required a lot of adjustment. Having become familiar with (and enthusiastic about) living with limited resources, and little or no 'waste culture'; we returned to an environment where people drove cars even short journeys, on their own, regardless of the environmental impact. The main form of entertainment, and source of knowledge, was the media and especially television which was now available all day long! That may sound rather judgmental but the transition from rural Indian life was quite extreme, and I had already reflected on many aspects of life in India which I felt could be usefully be copied in the UK in terms of improving our health. Much of this focused on putting less emphasis upon money and possessions and more on relationships with others and our surroundings.

One weekend I visited the newly founded Centre for Alternative Technology in Wales to get extra ideas about living 'with' rather than 'using' nature. With their help, I built a small Cretan windmill with canvas sails; of the style I had seen previously on the island of Mykonos in Greece during my gap year. It managed to power a few light bulbs with the help a redundant car generator. Despite using ash wood, which is flexible, strong and excellent for taking the strain of rotating sails; the beams snapped in strong wind after being transported up to Scotland. These were early days for wind power and using this technology was seen by most as eccentric, but now wind powered generators are very much in fashion. A pioneer in caring for the world's resources was Schumacher, who wrote his classic book 'Small is Beautiful' in 1972. His goal was not only to encourage conserving our planet's finite natural resources, but to foster close, localised and sustainable community living. This approach is now coming more into fashion for individuals and community groups but not yet substantially at a political level. His book was written during the mid-20th century drive for consumerism, throwaway possessions and debt.

My Serious Introduction to General Practice

The broad approach to medical care in general practice had appealed to me from early in my medical training. Temporary locum work during my sabbatical year reinforced this interest. My work in India involved a combination of general practice, primary and secondary care as well as preventive medicine, epidemiology and public health. However, when I returned to the UK, I realised that these specialties were spilt up with few overlapping responsibilities. The family care role of the general practitioner, when the patients had a personal doctor who knew their medical, social and family circumstances in detail, was disappearing. Home visits were avoided whenever possible and I felt surgeries were becoming run more like accident and emergency departments with the system encouraging doctors to see patients as illnesses. This, of course, does not stop the determined doctor from taking a more holistic approach, but it seemed to be becoming more difficult.

In contrast, practice in rural India was dependent on understanding the lifestyles and health needs of the people and their communities. Interestingly, now in the 21st century, this holistic approach seems be returning especially in rural areas where the general practitioner has the additional status of a general physician. Approaches to care such as acupuncture, chiropody, massage, aroma and music therapy, cognitive behavioural therapy, self-hypnosis and mindfulness are no longer branded as unscientific and of no proven value. In the meantime, hospital care has become mostly split into specialties where there is a need for very detailed expertise related to the highly technical and complicated investigations and treatments now available.

General Practice Training

I quickly found a one year training post in Bromsgrove which was 'home territory' since that was my local town during teenage years and where I went to school. Initially we stayed with my parents at their new house in the village of Shrawley near Worcester but through family contacts we then rented a small, newly built, farm cottage that was near to the practice. The cottage was next to the farm from where we collected daily supplies of unpasteurised milk as we had done in India. My desire to maintain self-sufficiency and environmentally friendly practices, that had been the 'norm' where we lived in India, was strong, and our small, previously uncultivated garden soon began to grow vegetables. We made dandelion root tea which had been a wartime drink replacing tea leaves, and could be mixed with dried chicory roots. It was a very long, hot and dry summer so when rain started, this prompted a glut of field mushrooms that meant we collected bucket loads and dried, froze, ate and gave away.

Although most of my work in India had been in primary care, the new Royal College of General Practitioners did not recognise this as being relevant to General Practice in the UK, so I was required to go through a registration process. This involved a one-year attachment to a recognised teaching practice plus weekly meetings with other trainees and trainers in the area.

I needed a car to be able to undertake house visits so bought a small, second hand, yellow rather sporty machine (which was somewhat out of character), from a friend of my sister. However, after bumping into another vehicle on a narrow road, I sold it to be replaced by a small fibre glass four wheeled Reliant Kitten which was very economical on petrol and did all I required. The accident was because I had not realised flashing lights towards oncoming vehicles in England is an invite for the other car to proceed - not as India where it is the reverse! However, I still carried out some home visits by bicycle, and on one visit about two miles from the surgery, I was simply asked to supply a sick certificate. The very pleasant woman felt so guilty that I was rewarded with numerous apologies, cups of tea and chocolate biscuits.

Bromsgrove had a district general hospital with various medical specialties but also a small cottage hospital run by the GPs. Interestingly, this included the accident and emergency services for the whole area. We performed minor surgery and had about 10 inpatient beds for patients who did not require special investigations or district hospital care. I 'lived in' when I was on-call. While most of the emergency patients had minor injuries, I witnessed several serious road accidents such as when a thirty year old business man died after presumably falling asleep and running into a motorway bridge; it was heartbreaking to be involved in caring initially for his nine year old daughter who had also been in the car. My sister was also admitted after a serious car accident while I was on duty; one of the other GPs attended to her.

Patients seen at the surgery were from both urban and rural backgrounds and our practice area encroached on the suburbs of Birmingham including residential areas that housed many workers from the Austin car factory in Longbridge. I discovered this was where much of the new living room furniture and large televisions sets advertised on television went to, usually on the 'never-never' otherwise called 'hire purchase'. In contrast, my family and friends tended to go for older and often second hand items even though their incomes were often greater, and this was because of a reluctance to take out loans. This was, as mentioned previously, around the time of the start of the age of con-sumerism made possible by the availability of easy credit.

Towards the end of my general practice year in Bromsgrove, I applied for a clinical lecturer post in infectious diseases with Glasgow University because it seemed to fit in with my previous experience and interests. I did not feel ready to commit myself to a full partnership in general practice and, at that time, part-time posts were hard to come by.

INFECTION AND IMPORTED DISEASES
IN GLASGOW

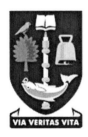

When I applied for the post of clinical lecturer in infectious diseases with Glasgow University, there was no obligation to complete a specified training programme for more senior hospital posts, and my application innocently consisted of half a page of hand written qualifications, appointments and hobbies. It now seems that even young school children are expected to start compiling a written and detailed 'curriculum vitae'! I have heard it suggested that parents should consider getting their very young children on the application list for their chosen schools or even golf clubs from birth! 'In the moment' knowledge, attitudes and abilities seem to be of secondary importance to a written record and may only be assessed in one-stop short interviews which can be a lottery. Training in how to put on a good 'act' or 'performance' at interviews is available which makes the whole procedure seem rather farcical. I wonder how many of those on interview panels get training in how to conduct themselves? At the Medical College in Vellore, interviews for medical school places took a week with careful counselling for both successful and unsuccessful candidates, which is another approach but time consuming. However, when I was appointed to a lecturer's post in Glasgow University (logo), my interview was relaxed and it was clear (despite my very brief CV) that my general medicine, infectious diseases and laboratory experience carried weight with the panel; perhaps in particular my time in India as a lecturer in medicine.

For the first 3 months I lived in the hospital while arrangements were made for the family to move north. This involved commuting back and forward to Worcestershire at weekends along the M6 and M5 motorways in my small Reliant Kitten car. It was not very sturdy in the wind, and once I stopped in the emergency carriageway in a gale to have the fiberglass door blown off when I opened it. Otherwise, it was reliable and very economical to run. The lecturer's post allowed me more freedom than being employed by the health service alone. While having daily and weekend clinical duties, I was able to focus on teaching and research with the guidance of our head of department, Professor Norman Grist. While I was based in a hospital, access to all the university facilities and links with other departments were possible as well as short sabbaticals at the head of department's discretion. I was able to return to CMCH in Vellore for 3 months at one stage.

Ruchill Hospital's History

The hospital was built as an isolation hospital at the beginning of the 20th century. Like many fever hospitals of that time, it was built on a hill where it was thought that fresh air and breezes would limit the spread of infection. As it was on a hill, the hospital needed a tall tower into which water was pumped and then distributed by gravity to the wards. This reminded me of similar systems in India when water was sometimes pumped up into a high concrete or metal containers from an enclosed well and then piped to individual houses replacing open wells and buckets except when the 'master' well was empty.

This was when our understanding of how infections are spread and could be prevented was far from complete, but there was recognition of the importance of avoiding person to person spread, a healthy environment and clean water.

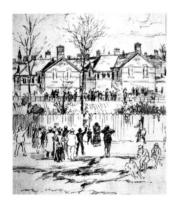 Also, during the first half of the 20th century, there were few effective antibiotic treatments, prophylactic medicines or vaccinations available. As an isolation hospital, Ruchill had high surrounding walls with glass concreted in along its top, to prevent people climbing over, and a manned security gate. In these hospitals relatives were not normally allowed onto the wards, to prevent the spread of infections, but may have been allowed into a special room where they could speak to a member of the ward staff who stood at a distance on a balcony or they could wave to the patients over the hospital walls (see drawing). Staff who had close contact with patients lived in a special accommodation building and also went into quarantine before they were allowed out for holidays into the wider community.

Since the hospital had a 'closed' community of staff, it had extensive grounds for recreation including a tennis court and croquet lawn. There was an orchard and vegetable garden within the grounds. The doctors' accommodation and nurses' home were substantial, with all meals provided; a recreation hall, library lounges and a billiard room - all still intact when I joined the staff. A rhubarb bed and many fruit trees still remained. While I was there, one of the junior doctors kept a small enclosed hive of bees in his bedroom, taking advantage of their pollen and nectar. The bees were allowed in and out along a tube through the window. While this seemed strange to some, as a bee keeper I could not see any health risks with this unless of course anyone intruded and started annoying them.

A magnificent stained glass window depicting the parable of the Good Samaritan was installed halfway up the main entrance staircase. When non-medical 'business managers' were being appointed to replace medical superintendents in the 1980s, the first manager decided that this window was inappropriate and 'made the staircase too dark'. He had it dismantled to be stored in a cellar. One can only surmise at his real motives, but it seemed at the time to relate to the health service downgrading humanitarian patient care to be replaced by a financially-focused agenda.

Originally the Hospital had more than 20 wards for infectious disease cases. By the 1980s when I joined the staff, it was down to four adult and one children's ward.

The hospital also housed the West of Scotland regional virus reference laboratory headed up by Professor

Norman Grist (pitured on the right - 'blanketing' grass to collect ticks on Arran in relation to lyme disease and louping ill), special bacteriology and parasitology facilities and importantly the Communicable Diseases Scotland Unit (CDSU). The CDS Unit was set up in the 1970s as a national rapid response, surveillance and epidemiology centre following a large outbreak of typhoid in Aberdeen due to infected corned beef having been imported from South America. This was before a similar public health

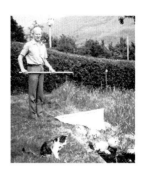

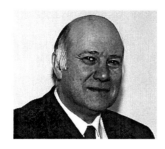

unit was set up in Colindale in London to serve other parts of the United Kingdom - Dr Dan Read was its founding director (pictured here). He oversaw the expansion of the unit through various reincarnations and throughout had a special interest in imported and travel related infections.

Other hospital departments included separate facilities for tuberculosis, a chest diseases unit, wards for care of the elderly and separate office accommodation for the University's infectious diseases and community health staff.

Patients with poliomyelitis, scarlet fever, smallpox, cholera and diphtheria all had separate wards allocated to them. Wooden and iron airtight boxes used intermittent negative pressure to allow patients with paralyzed respiratory muscles due to poliomyelitis to breath. They were used until positive pressure machines were introduced in the 1950s and 1960s. One advantage was that they did not require a tracheostomy, intubation or sedation and allowed the head to be free for normal eating, nose blowing etc.

A major advantage of this arrangement was that all the above wards, laboratories and departments dealing with infection were on one site and staff worked as a team. This meant issues relating to patients' illnesses and outbreaks, and also research topics could be easily discussed with colleagues at weekly case conferences or informally over lunch. It is no surprise that this multidisciplinary team approach made the Hospital into a leading centre, being among the first to recognise, for example, UK cases of legionnaire's disease, hantavirus infection, HIV infection, toxic shock, coxsackie virus related post-viral fatigue, antibiotic resistant staphylococci, tuberculous multi-drug resistance and anthrax relating to intravenous drug use.

Of special interest from a travel medicine perspective, was our identifying the first cases of legionnaire's disease outside of North America in tourists who had returned from Spain. We were able to trace the hotels where the infections had originated and that it was due to contaminated water cooled air-conditioning and shower systems. This episode triggered a number of research projects and led to a European-wide immediate reporting system to allow early identification of outbreaks.

A Selection of Clinical Experiences

During this period, the reasons for admission to hospital were rapidly changing with more and improved vaccines, greater awareness of food and water contamination which allowed preventive procedures to be put in place. Also, new effective antimicrobials were being discovered that could be used in general practice and reduce the need for hospital care.

- Tetanus and diphtheria where already rare due to vaccination schedules for children and measles was already becoming less common due to vaccination started in the 1970s.

- Mumps and rubella cases fell when a combined vaccine became available. An exception was whooping cough that had returned due to a media scare about the safety of its vaccine which was eventually shown to be unfounded.

- Cases of chickenpox, usually more severe in adults, continued. Its vaccine was, and still is, only used in exceptional circumstances. Complications and the pain of shingles become less common with the availability of an effective antiviral drug although it took some time before general practitioners were persuaded to use it early in the illness.

- Smallpox was declared eradicated worldwide in the 1970s but until then we were entrusted with immunising medical students during their training in infectious diseases at the hospital. Large stocks of smallpox vaccine were kept in case the smallpox virus became used for germ warfare and the rumour was that we were targeted for one of the first nuclear bomb strikes if war was to break out! I saw facial scars from previous smallpox in India which was one of the last countries to achieve eradication.

- In children, common problems were croup, bronchiolitis and diarrhoea. It was quite late on when it was recognised that early rehydration is the key to successful treatment for diarrhoea. Simplistically many of the public still thought fluids given by mouth would just pass straight through and make the diarrhoea worse as was still the case in India. Diarrheoal illness in adults was common although improvements in poultry management have made salmonella infections much less common.

- In adults, pneumonia, meningitis, hepatitis, rashes due to viral and bacterial infections and glandular fever were common. Many patients with headaches were admitted because of the possibility that they could be due to meningitis or encephalitis. Jaundice from the various causes of hepatitis was common and tests to identify types A, B, C, D and E were available from the 1980-1990s.

- Diarrhoeal illnesses contracted abroad were sometimes due to unusual causes like cholera, giardiasis and amoebiasis rarely now contracted in the UK. When fever was present, malaria and typhoid had to be quickly excluded. More unusual imported infections included, intestinal worms and leprosy.

- When serious, untreatable, haemorrhagic diseases such

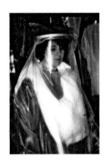

as Lassa and Ebola fever were first recognised in Africa we were designated as a centre with special expertise and a high standard isolation unit was built. This 'Trexler unit' (below) had been designed by a veterinarian for use when nursing animals with diseases thought at the time to be highly contagious. As it turned out, we only used it when medical students volunteered to be patients so as to give staff practice in managing the unit and its equipment.

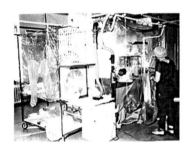

- I remember one 'plague scare', when we had journalists waiting outside the wards looking for stories and pictures - the patient involved had influenza but had become feverish on a plane from India where an outbreak was occurring. A stewardess raised the alarm and the media somehow got to know about the situation before the patient arrived at the hospital! We now know more about these newly recognised infections, and there is generally less of a sense of panic when suspect cases occur, and there are well-defined procedures for management.

- Media interest in infections is unpredictable and can take up a lot of time - we used to consider Friday afternoons were a time for media calls from journalists looking for last minute Sunday newspaper stories. Once, I spoke to a journalist who had been given the task of writing an article about malaria in relation to one of our patients, whose relatives had informed the newspaper editor. She clearly knew next to nothing about the disease and had not done any background reading. I correctly suspected I was going to be quoted by name, probably inaccurately, and my comments displayed in a melodramatic manner. Usually single events like this resulted in many more calls from other media sources for several days afterwards. Later, I attended a course on coping with media enquiries run by an ex-journalist, which was very helpful - 'First ask what they want to talk about and then say you will ring them back' was very sound advice giving you time to prepare what you wanted to say and not get distracted onto other subjects.

HIV Infection and AIDS

When the human immunodeficiency virus (HIV) appeared on the scene there was much anxiety involved in caring for these young patients because, although it had the features of being an infection, we did not know what the cause was, or how it was spread. We recognised that it was often related to homosexuality although one of our first patients was a young woman who had contracted the infection through heterosexual exposure in Greece. Sharing needles among intravenous drug users, which was rife in certain areas of Glasgow, was quickly recognised as another route of infection. We did not know if it was spread by means other than sex or blood. I remember, while taking a teaching ward round, knocking over a patient's urine bottle which was under his bed and afterwards spending some time disinfecting my shoes in case I would take infection home to my family - as it turns out now this would have been a most unlikely source of infection.

Subsequently we were involved in identifying the responsible organism, establishing reliable diagnostic tests, working on prevention strategies, especially within the gay and drug using communities, and being involved in public education programmes. Edinburgh had a bigger problem than Glasgow where drug users tended to share needles in groups of two or three. In Edinburgh larger groups congregated in 'shooting galleries' as a social event, and passed the heroin around using the same syringe and needle.

Ruchill Hospital was one of the first centres in the UK to set up needle exchange services and methadone drug replacement in an attempt to prevent injecting and sharing of needles. Both these initiatives were very controversial and the hospital gates were picketed for many months by local residents who thought our prevention strategies encouraged drug use. Maybe there was limited truth in this, but our focus was on prevention of this new and terrible disease that was rapidly killing many young people through a slow and inexorable death. The early epidemic years were comparable to the days when many young people died from tuberculosis before the days of antibiotics.

We had a special HIV ward for the most seriously ill that provided terminal care. However, all this changed about 8 years later when effective drugs that could be given in combination (multidrug therapy) were found to give long-term control, although not elimination, of the virus. The vast majority of AIDS patients then lost their symptoms, put on weight and stopped getting the opportunistic secondary infections that killed them. 'Opportunistic' infection included severe candidiasis, cytomegalovirus, toxoplasmosis, cryptosporidiosis, pneumocystis and some forms of tuberculosis, were commonly around but only cause serious illness in those with an inadequate immune response.

Those identified with early HIV infections usually now remain well with adequate and early anti-HIV treatment although some still present late with complications unaware that they were infected many years previously. In India both the arrival of HIV infection and then subsequent cases was about 5-10 years behind the UK, so these early experiences in Glasgow were of great value when helping with education and management programmes in India as part of our Indo-UK linked programme discussed later.

Teaching

Undergraduate teaching was a highlight for me. Infectious and tropical diseases looked at from a global perspective were subjects that seemed to catch students' imagination and I find this is still the case. Many are strongly motivated by humanitarian career goals, focusing on people in countries with poor living conditions and medical services.

My teaching responsibilities at Ruchill included series of 6-week courses for 4th year medical students. These started with slides and discussions where I used a lot of my pictures from Africa and India as well as photographs taken in Ruchill's wards themselves. We then went on ward rounds in small groups. Many of the students I now meet from time to time as fully qualified doctors, often they know me but I may only know their faces. With three colleagues, I wrote a book called 'Diseases of Infection'. It became very popular, in part I believe, because the approach was very practical, being written by clinicians with input from the related laboratory and public health staff present on the hospital campus.

Later, we began a tropical diseases course so as to enable postgraduate students to take a Diploma in Tropical Medicine examination in London. This began in an informal way, taking advantage of expertise, enthusiasm and overseas experience available both in the University, Glasgow hospitals and general practice who gave their time freely.

A significant amount of time was spent writing articles, preparing lectures and epidemiological research and it was during the 1980s that personal computers were introduced. The most dramatic change was the move away from using mechanical typewriters. Prior to this when any changes or corrections were necessary either the whole page had to be retyped or 'Typex' (a simple white paint applied with a small brush) used to obscure the error so they could be typed over. This was a 'godsend' to both the secretaries and authors who then had so much more freedom to write drafts and not feel guilty about making alterations.

Health Service and University Politics Resulting in Major Changes

By the year 2000, all the hospital departments in Ruchill were split up and rehoused in different sites around Glasgow as part of a reorganisation exercise. Before this happened, the 'Communicable Disease Scotland Unit' had became the 'Scottish Centre for Infection and Environmental Health' - later to become 'Health Protection Scotland'. It is now confined to managing outbreaks and giving national advice on disease prevention. It has no direct clinical input except in terms of receiving disease notifications and laboratory reports and is based in an office block in the centre of the city. Responsibility for undergraduate infectious disease teaching was transferred to the University's public health department and the microbiology laboratories to other hospitals. From a teaching perspective, this meant students no longer saw a broad cross section of common infectious diseases in a multidisciplinary setting.

It was very difficult for many of us to see logic in these changes, but the decisions were out of our hands and taken by the Scottish Health Department, the University's Medical Faculty and the Glasgow Health Board. There seemed to be a perception that infections were becoming a thing of the past since we now had adequate vaccinations for prevention and antibiotics for treatment. This misconception was already clearly visible to those of us involved on the 'shop floor'. For example, newly recognised emerging and re-emerging infections were already spreading rapidly around the world as a result of the new ease and speed of travel. Also, widespread antimicrobial drug resistance and hospital-acquired infections were appearing. Many of us felt policy-making detached from front-line involvement meant that there would be a risk, for example, of both over and under-estimating the seriousness of various infections. This could lead policy makers to react more to media pressure and fears of litigation than to scientific evidence when making important public health decisions. Convincing the public about the importance of preventive measures, including vaccinations, when those giving the advice have little or no experience of the illnesses involved, would become more difficult and sometimes loose credence. An example of this is when measles is displayed as a lethal disease - it can be, but this is very rare in a well-nourished population and when antibiotics are available to treat complications. Older members of the public already know this having had the disease themselves as children. I saw this difference in mortality patterns in India when the death rate in villages could be as high as 25% during epidemics while 'just down the road' among hospital staff serious complications were very rare. The first inactivated measles virus vaccine also caused serious side-effects but now there is a live attenuated vaccine that seems safe but does need booster doses in adult life which was not appreciated initially.

Uncertainty, All Change and the Need for Health Advice for Travellers

My university lecturer post was tenured, which meant it could not be terminated without my agreement, but I was told by the Dean at the time that I would have no chance of promotion and I should leave. The reality was that the integrated multidisciplinary approach to managing infections that I enjoyed, had disappeared anyway.

Amidst all this uncertainty, I applied for a general practice partnership in Galashiels in the Scottish Border region. I was offered the post but turned it down after much heart wrenching. It was in a two-doctor practice that had refused the opportunity of joining other local practitioners in a new modern health centre. I thought there was potential personality issues involved in this decision over which I would have little control, and I would also have been asked to do most of the nights on-call without any locum help. However, shortly after, I was offered a consultant post with Health Protection Scotland which involved national responsibility for surveillance and the prevention of tropical and travel related diseases. I also retained 2 days a week clinical work on the infectious diseases wards, and was given an honorary role as a senior university lecturer.

It is interesting to reflect that, without these upheavals, I would probably not have had the opportunity to participate in the development of the new speciality: travel medicine. These services were initially a simple response, by default, to the huge increase in demand for advice from overseas travellers during the 1970s and 1980s. This had come about, as explained later, because high speed air transport had become available for travellers and business people with the creation of wide-bodied 'jumbo jet' aircraft. Being responsible for this advice service was a major challenge, as the demand rapidly outstripped the resources available. Those managing the health services had not yet recognised there was an unavoidable and growing need for the NHS to become computerised. As there was no other centre in the UK (NHS or private) with the facilities or interest in providing travel health advice, I found myself regularly taking more than 100 phone calls a day from medical and nursing colleagues as well as the general public who had been given our phone number by their general practitioners.

The further development of travel medicine services is described later with an explanation of how a comprehensive service was developed in Scotland with continually updated information being made available for the public and their healthcare advisors, training in providing services and with secondary level referrals being available at NHS infectious disease units. In England and Wales especially, private clinics where patients had to pay, for example, for their appointments plus any vaccines or medications began to develop as an alternative.

How far travel medicine should be an NHS responsibility is still debated with private clinics arguing their case - some provide excellent services but they are generally unregulated. Opponents say that it can be difficult for private clinics to provide comprehensive care and advice when they do not know details of the traveller's medical history like their general practitioners. These details can be very important for those with existing illnesses such as diabetes, heart and lung disease, or others on regular medications as is often the case with the elderly. Also, contracting diseases abroad can be very expensive for the NHS on the traveller's return, and include GP and hospital consultations, medications, admissions and even intensive care for serious illnesses such typhoid, malignant malaria and rabies. There is also the risk of spread of infections after travellers come home, including hepatitis A, typhoid, diphtheria, meningitis, influenza, tuberculosis, HIV infection and haemorrhagic fevers such as Lassa and Ebola.

CONTINUING INDIAN
COLLABORATION

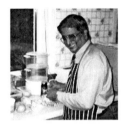 As explained previously, my lecturer's appointment at the Christian Medical College and Hospital was formally with Madras University since CMCH was, at that time, not an independent medical school. This meant that I built up connections with the University and especially their Virology Department in the Postgraduate Institute of Basic Medical Sciences (PIBMS) in Chennai through Professor Thyagarajan and Dr Suniti Solomon. After return to UK these links became much closer because of common interests in hepatitis B and later in the management of HIV infection.

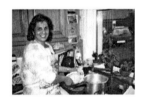

The Postgraduate Institute
of Basic Medical Sciences Council

Hepatitis B and the Phyllanthus Story

A collaborative educational link, supported by the British Council, was established between the infectious disease unit in Glasgow and the PIBMS around 1985. We had annual exchange visits in each direction for doctors and nurses that facilitated a wide variety of symposia and research projects.

170

The research component initially focused on epidemio-logical studies of the various forms of viral hepatitis. This led to educational programmes among medical staff as well as at risk groups, such as blood transfusion recipients and injecting drug users.

Part of this work included a programme to study the effectiveness of a herbal remedy for jaundice made from a small wild plant, phyllanthus amarus that is widespread throughout India. I had become aware of this plant when 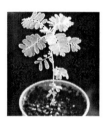 working in the villages while at CMCH Vellore since it was common practice to collect this plant, boil it, make it into a small soft pellet and then give it to the jaundiced patient to swallow. This was a very long-standing local practice that suggested that there could be some real beneficial effect.

Initially, scientifically valid studies with patients were carried out in India with confirmatory blood tests being performed in Glasgow that suggested phyllanthus had a significant effect in eliminating hepatitis B virus from their blood. We carried out some small additional studies in Scotland and I brought over some seeds and grew plants in one of the greenhouses in Glasgow's botanical gardens. Amusingly, the pods released their seeds explosively so new plants started growing through the greenhouse - the keeper was very understanding.

On one occasion I brought 200 capsules containing phyllanthus back to Scotland in my suitcase to carry out a local trial. The suitcase was damaged in transit and delayed during a change over flight in Paris. This meant customs officers in Glasgow got very excited when my damaged suitcase containing lots of herbs and unidentified capsules arrived the next day. I was fortunately able to show them the relevant import certificates!

Eventually, further research in the UK was not possible because regulations were introduced that did not allow trials of herbal remedies with NHS patients when the active chemical principal had not been determined. This seemed a strange approach when so many effective modern medicines were originally derived from plants which had been known, for many years previously, to have beneficial effects. This new legislation means that it is only large drug companies with the money to carry out such studies can be involved, and that the patent would belong to them and not the person(s) responsible for initiating the idea.

The Y.R. Gaitonde Centre for AIDS Research, Care and Education

I was privileged to observe and support the establishment of the YRG Centre from its inception. Very close friendships have developed over the years. Dr Suniti Solomon, was originally a consultant virologist at the Madras Medical Hospital and was the first person in India to identify HIV positive sex workers at a time when the infection was not thought to be, or going to be, a problem in India. She had already been involved in our Indo-UK link project on hepatitis. As the pandemic arrived in India about 5-10 years after the UK, the British Council asked us to switch the focus of our projects from hepatitis to HIV. We were able to share ten year's experience in helping set up prevention programmes and later give guidance on the care of patients with AIDS. The YRG centre was named after Suniti's husband, a cardiac surgeon, who donated funds to help it get established.

Suniti recognised that there were going to be big problems regarding awareness, counselling, diagnosis and care. There was considerable prejudice against those infected, and denial that HIV would become widespread. In reality there are now more HIV positive people in India (about 2-3% of the population of more than 2 billion) than in the whole of sub-Saharan Africa with its smaller total population.

At that time, patients were frequently tested for HIV infection without their permission when they attended hospitals for other reasons, and if found positive were discharged and denied any further care. Suniti established a centre in 1994 for testing and counselling these and other worried people in a private house that she rented. This expanded to provide a few inpatient beds and later the whole service moved to a wing in a voluntary non-governmental hospital that had previously been used for leprosy patients.

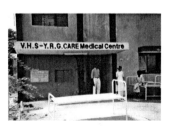

Now, 20 years later, the YRG is a very important

counselling, research, care and training centre with a national and international reputation. Professional sex work is common in India and is often carried out openly, although in some states this is illegal. Any sense of blame or shame was formally attached only to the women not their male 'customers' and sex workers were often 'rounded up' and put in jail for short periods of time. Drug use through snuffing or inhaling is common while injecting occurs, but is rarer.

Truck drivers and their young assistants are at particular risk of HIV infection through liaising with professional sex workers when they are away from home for long periods, sometimes 4-6 weeks at a time. Awareness of the risk among young women, who frequently marry men in their mid-twenties, is now improving and pre-marriage counselling and testing is becoming more common. Using unsterile needles and other medical equipment remains a serious problem when disposables cannot be afforded and efficient sterilisers are not available. Disposing of sharps by putting them out as rubbish often means they are scavenged, sold on and reused.

Educational and Research Activities Conducted through the British Council Link

During this Link programme I visited Chennai annually for more than 15 years, often with colleagues from Glasgow, and there were the same frequent visits of Indian staff to Glasgow. In both centres, we set up educational symposia for various groups of physicians and nurses. In India we also held meetings for community groups in schools and colleges and for the media. As well as looking at preventive, social and clinical aspects of HIV infection, we included symposia on ethical issues which highlighted the differing approaches and

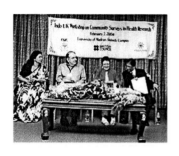

emphases necessary, depending upon the cultural and occupational backgrounds of those involved. Over the years, these meetings included evenings for the public at British Council Offices and courses in many hospitals in Tamil Nadu and elsewhere in South India and the Andaman Islands where there is an HIV link with fishermen coming ashore from Thailand. Thailand was one of the first countries in Southeast Asia to recognise it had a serious HIV problem.

In Glasgow, we held hepatitis B and AIDS seminars for our Indian visitors together with local medical and nursing staff. We visited wards and outreach centres, such as pharmacies, where needle exchanges had been set up for intravenous drug users. Eight nurses came over on one occasion, when a programme for them on 'universal' precautions to prevent the spread of HIV in hospitals had been setup in collaboration with Caledonian University. (They did not take well to Scottish food so they also enjoyed doing their own cooking and exploring the shops.) In 2004 we held a day long seminar on ethical issues relating to the diagnosis and care of patients with HIV infection to which staff contributed both from Glasgow and from India. Following this, an ongoing annual ethics symposium was setup by the YRG centre in Chennai which has attracted both national and international speakers.

Educational efforts in the community have involved counselling truck drivers at the roadside and education for HIV drug users and sex 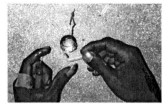 workers. One awareness exercise was to set up a stall at a regular highway rest point for truck drivers. Sex workers would usually wait in huts a few miles beyond the restaurant for clients. Our stall gave a chance to discuss the risk and how AIDS is spread with the drivers and demonstrate how to use condoms using plastic models. I wonder how this would go down on the high street in Glasgow - probably we would end up arrested!

We visited a nearby tourist resort where a local Roman Catholic priest was involved in a similar exercise with sex workers. The women would come out to the resort from Chennai in buses and had arrangements with local hotels who provided rooms for them to carry out their trade. Similarly, we held workshops with groups of sex workers in the city itself that were both useful and entertaining. Many of these sex workers were from rural areas and been disowned by their families when their husbands had either left them or died. They usually had young children and so began sex work to earn money as their apparent only option to provide food for they families, (unlike in the UK where many sex workers trade to fund costly drug addiction problems). I remember a humorous discussion over whether it would be safer to use two condoms at the same time instead of one! There was often a refreshing openness when discussing these issues, more so than in the UK. Among young nurses in hospitals there was usually a widely held view that one partner and one marriage was the only way forward. Unfortunately, this approach does not take fully into account issues such as when widows have no family or social support and feel they have no alternative to prostitution to provide for themselves and their children. This educational work over many years relating to Hepatitis and HIV infection and supported by the British Council was acknowledged when I was awarded a Doctorate (DSc) from Madras University in 2001.

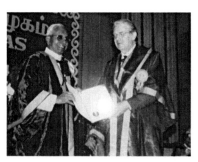

Throughout this time, whenever possible, I combined my trips with a visit to CMCH in Vellore keeping up friendships especially with Sara and Suranjan Battacharji, attending ward rounds, giving some talks and informally meeting junior staff. As time went on Sara moved from work mainly in the villages to focus on services for the urban poor in Vellore town where she established a pioneering centre providing low cost effective medical care. Suranjan

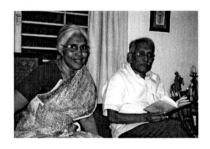

throughout specialized in rehabilitation surgery and developing low cost equipment such as splits and wheel chairs for the many people who had longterm injuries to limbs and spine from accidents and falls - later he served for 5 years as director of the institution. Both are inspirational in showing what can be done through hard work and compassion to provide excellent services for those who would otherwise miss out through poverty or other personal circumstances from access to the best of medical care.

Experiences Travelling with Colleagues in India

When revisiting Chennai and Vellore, I often travelled with medical or nursing colleagues. This was a mixed blessing since some of my companions, despite explanation beforehand, clearly had great difficulty in adapting to the fact that going to India is not like going on a package holiday to the Mediterranean. These trips meant I had company travelling, which I enjoyed, but there were times when there were obvious 'culture shock' difficulties, and I felt somewhat responsible and was occasionally openly blamed for not arranging things better. Examples of this were when we missed flights due to overbooking or cancellation. There was no way we could be informed about this in advance, it was before mobile phones and the unreliable landlines made telephone confirmations of flights difficult. The normal practice, back in the 1980s and 1990s, was to go personally to the airline offices, usually in Chennai, and confirm return flights face-to face with airline staff. This was impossible if you were staying outside the city and sometimes special couriers were employed to make the confirmations which could involve one or two days travelling - alternatively we could arrange to spend the final days of a trip 'in town' ourselves.

Appropriate dress was a common problem since it was difficult to convince some female colleagues in advance that, when it is hot, it is usual to wear light airy clothes rather than to go around, seeming to the locals, to be half naked. Scanty swimming costumes in hotel swimming pools inevitably invited an audience mostly made up of staff and day visitors. Sometimes companions took duty-free alcohol out with them, which could be embarrassing since drinking alcohol at the time was usually only done in private, in hotel bars and by men.

On one trip I travelled with a group of about twenty previous travel medicine diploma students and tutors who wished to gain 'on the ground' experience in India. With help from my Indian colleagues, we tried to make the trip as authentic and interesting as possible avoiding five star hotels and luxury coaches and visiting government and rural hospitals, water treatment and sewage works. Meat is not widely eaten in South India. Part of the reason is linked to religious practices, but it is possibly also because, without refrigeration, meat goes rotten quickly. However, some of the group decided that they needed a change from vegetarian spicy food and went to a nearby Chinese restaurant for chicken chow mein. Nearly all of them developed dysentery the next day and one ended up being repatriated. The message must be: as far as possible, eat as the educated locals do because they don't wish to get ill either! Despite having their travel medicine diploma, 90% of this group had illnesses varying from dysentery to sunburn. Some had influenza contracted on the journey out and one young woman was repatriated suffering 'culture shock', made worse after meeting a rat in her bathroom.

After helping to conduct an HIV workshop, our onward journey from Chennai provided an interesting experience. Officially, planes were only allowed to take off with a limited number of passengers because the runway was too short for a full load. However, in resourceful fashion, many of the empty seats were used to carry sacks of mangos and other fruits and vegetables so the weight of the plane was not significantly reduced. The runway was on a slight downward slope and at the top there was a roundabout allowing planes to set off uphill and at the top, without stopping, circle round to develop a starting speed of maybe around 50mph. This allowed the planes to take off before running across a busy highway!

TRAVEL MEDICINE AND
GLOBAL HEALTH COMES OF AGE

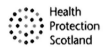 As described previously, during the 1980s I had been appointed to a consultant post with Health Protection Scotland (HPS and originally the Communicable Diseases Scotland Unit) at the time when Glasgow University abolished its academic infectious diseases department. I was given a national responsibility for surveillance and prevention of imported infections while retaining 2 days a week clinical work on the infectious diseases wards and in outpatients, which included the establishment of the first dedicated travel clinic in Scotland for complicated referrals for General Practice.

In addition to earlier travel experiences like hitchhiking around Europe, my exchange period as a student in Zimbabwe and time spent in India, working in this role with HPS allowed me additional opportunities for short visits overseas while continuing my research and education links with Chennai and Vellore. I undertook a number of short working visits to South Africa, New Zealand, Italy, Norway, Thailand, HongKong and Singapore mostly for research or education reasons or to support local or regional travel medicine societies most of which were in their infancy.

This was also the time when the International Society of Travel Medicine (ISTM) was established which gave me the opportunity to attend their regular conferences as well as contribute to the ISTM committee as editor of their newsletter for members.

A few years after I formally began work with Health Protection Scotland, the clinical department of Infection moved to Gartnavel General Hospital in Glasgow. This meant that my responsibilities were split between two sites geographically, about 3 miles apart. Since most infectious disease referrals at the time were for acute illnesses, my ability to be a consultant 'on the spot' for admissions and for follow up became impractical. I was still able however, to continue running pre- and post-travel clinics, and arrange admissions when necessary under the care of other consultants. I was uncomfortable about this detachment from patient care, and this was one of the reasons I felt the need later to leave Health Protection Scotland several years before my formal 'retirement' date. I returned to general practice in a part-time role while continuing an involvement with travel medicine through Deanship of the new Faculty of Travel Medicine, teaching with the University and supporting the British Travel Health Association (all described later).

Over this period, I was becoming increasingly disturbed by the competitive and business orientated approach to health care which was creeping into the National Health Service during the 1970s and 1980s - the end of medicine as a profession as my father described it. This was very obvious within Health Protection Scotland. Instead of being able to focus on promoting health and preventing or managing disease, we were being instructed to continually prove our worth in economic and business management terms. We had to produce annual business and strategic plans, record all we did, even supply confirmation of when we were thanked by patients for helping them. We were required to document the hours we worked including relevant out-of-hours activities, and undertake appraisals with colleagues who may have little or no knowledge of the day-to-day work involved in our specialty. This involved completing numerous forms that we suspected were rarely understood or looked at seriously by those to whom they were submitted. The focus of this exercise was on the prestige of the unit in the eyes of health service managers entrusted to look at the 'bigger picture' and prioritise resources.

Of course, compassion and caring for other individuals cannot be evaluated effectively by data collection and statistics but we were made to think that 'qualitative' activities were unimportant or even irrelevant. What I found most distasteful was feeling an obligation to 'show off' which encouraged exaggeration of those aspects of our work that we thought would please our business managers. 'Standing on a table and shouting out how wonderful we are' was, and I hope still is, obscene and foreign to a very large proportion of healthcare staff.

The Birth of Travel Medicine as a Speciality

Since the 1970s there had been a huge increase in overseas air travel for both holiday and business purposes. The increase in the numbers of those leaving the UK for overseas has risen from around 5 million in the 1970s to over 60 million in 2010. The other big change is that from the 1980s, emails, internet and mobile phone technology has meant that the days of working abroad for years at a time, with little or no contact with those back home, have gone. We are surely in a communications revolution and are still learning how to adjust our attitudes and lifestyles accordingly. These dramatic changes can be difficult to appreciate for those less than around 30-40 years of age who have known nothing else. Similarly those older may be unable to understand why younger people take these changes for granted when they are all dependent upon reliable technology and secure electricity supplies!

I usually say my involvement in travel medicine at this time came about by default, since it was in response to the immediate need, when there were no other reliable or comprehensive resources on health advice available in the UK for either travellers or their advisors. It was one of those 'here is a need, can you help?' situations. Looking back, I suppose my quite extensive exploration and adventure travelling from a young age, my infectious and tropical disease and epidemiological training and experience as well as my time in Africa and India, put me in good stead to become involved. I would like to think my experience and fascination with how we relate to the natural environment also shaped my approach to the subject.

Previously, health advice for those going abroad was only available anecdotally from those with previous experience and there was little in the way of definitive advice. Medical officers of health who ran yellow fever vac-

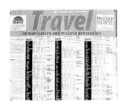

cination centres issued international vaccination certificates, but medical officer posts were abolished in the 1970s and replaced by public health consultants who had a much broader remit and many had little or no infectious disease or vaccination training, let alone overseas experience. There was a gap in expertise that needed to be filled because of the new and increasing demand from the travelling public and their healthcare advisors, mostly general practitioners. The vaccine manufactures began to fill this gap in information by supplying charts that gave very simplified information on what vaccine were recommended for different countries. This guidance was usually grossly oversimplified and did not involve what we now call a thorough risk assessment for each individual traveller in relation to their intended itinerary and likely activities.

After publishing an article on malaria in immigrants returning to visit their families abroad in the British Medical Journal, I was invited by the journal's editor to write a practical handbook on health issues related to travel. I called it the 'The ABC of Healthy Travel'. It focused on the needs of general practitioners and practice nurses who were giving advice to their travelling patients, but was in a from that could also be useful to the lay public. It went to 5 editions and eventually was taken over by the advent of TRAVAX on-line.

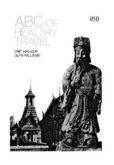

As explained previously, I already had a special interest in the health of travellers and now created a continually updated information resource using an 'index' card for every country in the world which could be 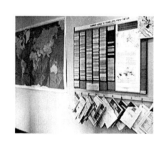 referred to by those taking phone calls. Since there was no other such service in the UK, the numbers of calls quickly became unmanageable and I was personally sometimes taking over 100 calls a day on top of my university, ward and

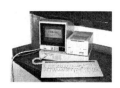 outpatient commitments. Callers were from all over the UK and many were from the public who had been told to ring by their general practice receptionists. We did not encourage the public to contact us since we were not able to make detailed risk assessments on the phone and, more importantly, did not have the responsibility for prescribing or administering their medications or vaccines. So, when telephone based communications technology such as CEEFAX arrived we took advantage of this, followed 5-10 years later by the internet. The databases have become very widely used both in the UK and abroad in other English speaking countries as the public Fit-For-Travel and the professional TRAVAX websites. A major difficulty was that general practices were only just beginning to install computers in their premises and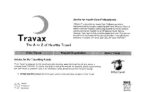

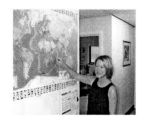

many did not know how to use websites and needed training. Also, initially computers and the software they used were often unreliable and this took some years to improve to an acceptable level.

Vital members of our travel medicine team at this early stage were Fiona Genasi and Lorna Boyne shown here in the travel clinic.

An interesting challenge at this time was creating an inventory for the European Commission of the nature of Travel Medicine services in the European Union countries. This was a major task and

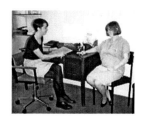

one of the most important outcomes was getting to know, in these early days, individuals in each country who were involved. Creation of this professional network has been

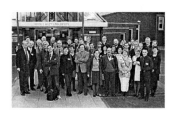

invaluable in subsequent years. This photograph was taken at a meeting in Edinburgh of all the participants to discuss the results and help develop the final report.

The Importance of Considering the Environment

With my longstanding interest in man's relationship to nature, I was particularly interested in how travel health risks are closely related to our behaviour, especially when in countries and environments with which we are unfamiliar. To avoid illness, a greater understanding is needed by the traveller of how infections are spread, how serious they might be and, for example, how sudden climate changes can have serious health consequences and when accidents are more likely.

This knowledge is needed so that travellers can adjust their activities and ingrained habits so as to try and stay healthy. Particularly when in countries where government and local authorities do not take away from individuals much of the responsibility for preventing illness through health and safety regulations. Also how we use modern day travel facilities has a major impact on our environment now we have come to rely on polluting and finite energy sources.

Travel Medicine Education

Soon we realised that supplying information alone was not sufficient and that professionals using the on-line services needed not only training in how to both use the computers, but also in how to interpret the information for their patients and in particular how to make detailed risk assessments. The 'ABC of Healthy Travel' was helpfully distributed to many practices by one of the drug companies for us because getting monies for this purpose from the health service was like 'getting blood out of a stone'! The same company also provided us with the resources to employ and train a nurse which was the first time I had been given full-time support.

We then setup two-day courses in risk assessment for doctors and nurses. These courses were very popular but only served our local area. Trained teachers were needed throughout the country to run similar courses and eventually one of the students from our Diploma course took over these courses and conducted them at a national level. Other companies also offered to help but we had to tread carefully because some of them understandably wanted us to focus mainly on the need for vaccines that they manufactured.

The Travel Medicine Diploma

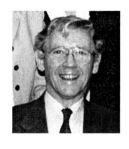

Because of this need for a higher level of training for those interested in the subject and those who wanted to teach, in 1995 a one-year distance learning Diploma course leading to an optional MSc was established in collaboration between Health Protection Scotland and Glasgow University. The late Cameron Lockie (above), a General Practitioner from Stratford-upon-Avon, undertook a sabbatical period in London to develop the course curriculum and became one of the first course tutors.

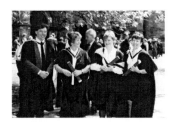

This is a photograph of some of the first Diploma/MSc students.

Medical and nursing schools have been very slow to include these basic skills into their national curricula and some think private medical companies should be the ones to give travel health advice since travel is not an illness. Others believe we have a national 'health' service not a 'disease' service and therefore have a responsibility for prevention and it is also a money saver when travellers don't come home ill. Many of 700 or so of those who have since completed the Diploma course have become experts in the specialty both in the UK and in other countries such as Australia, New Zealand, Canada and South Africa.

Early on during one of these Diploma courses over an evening dinner (or perhaps in the pub afterwards if I remember correctly) the idea of a British Travel Health Association (BTHA), later to become the British Global and Travel Health Association (BGTHA) was born. This Association has since then organised annual conferences, published a biennial journal and facilitated networking for travel health practitioners throughout the UK.

A Return to Part-time General Practice

I decided to retire a few years earlier than need be from my joint consultant post with Greater Glasgow Health Board and Health Protection Scotland in order to help set up a Faculty of Travel Medicine in the Glasgow Royal College. The Faculty's success suggests the timing was right for this initiative. This released me from the business, strategic and financial planning that had become a responsibility for doctors after the health service was being converted into a business during the end of the 20th century. My father had warned me about this many years previously in the 1970s, when doctors started to be paid a basic salary plus overtime, which he rightly foresaw was the start of the end of medicine as a full-time professional vocation.

This early retirement also gave me the opportunity to return to part-time general practice patient care. It had been becoming harder to continue with any clinical work since Health Protection Scotland was progressively becoming a public health domain where any clinical role was discouraged. I was not comfortable with this separation of roles for reasons that I hope I have made clear in previous chapters.

I joined a practice in Balfron, a small village near my home, where the two partners had managed to retain the traditional family practice structure with, for example, open surgeries every day and home visits for elderly patients in need. This holistic approach seems easier to retain in rural areas than in cities where health centres have become very large and run more as an outpatient style of service with appointments being the rule whenever possible and home visits are discouraged. Balfron practice gave me a real sense of being part of the local community and the work definitely had a 'Dr Finlay's case book' feel about it but with all the modern facilities and trimmings. For example, many doctors don't like to be friends with their patients and avoid meeting them socially but I found this sort of relationship rewarding and it was inevitable since the practice was in a village I knew. We had a dispensing pharmacy next door and this was a mutually beneficial way of working together for the benefit of patients, doctors and the pharmacist. Increasingly pharmacists are taking on a diagnostic and treatment roles for many minor illnesses, and I felt this worked well especially since the surgery and pharmacy were next door to each other and cross-referrals were easy to arrange.

The most difficult aspect I found was not always being able to review patient's acute problems myself on a daily basis since I was part-time and there was often a 'what if?' feeling at the end of surgeries. This however, was not a major problem because I could reliably pass on important follow-up issues to the other partners.

Balfron is about 18 miles from Glasgow and is one of about 10 villages situated just where the Scottish Central Lowlands reach the West Coast Highlands. Balfron was seen as a central village with the region's fire station, high school for secondary level pupils, the main post office, police station and a bank. The bulk of our patients were either in families where one or more members were commuters to Glasgow or Stirling, farmers, connected in some other way to the land and/or involved in local small businesses. As a result, the medical problems encountered included a wide range of conditions similar to those living in cities, as well as those related to rural pursuits. Attitudes to illness were very varied: some patients attending surgery for minor ailments, while others coming for advice only after they had tried a whole range of personal remedies. If a farmer called for a home visit it was sensible to drop everything and 'run' because a serious problem was likely. It was a privilege to be part of this community and I made many new friends of both colleagues and patients.

Establishing a Faculty of Travel Medicine

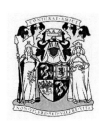

The Faculty of Travel Medicine was established in 2007 within the Royal College of Physicians and Surgeons in Glasgow, where the normal route of entry was by examination. I was appointed as the first Dean. The College was already multidisciplinary and including travel medicine within its remit was relatively straightforward. The only obstacle, which was at the time revolutionary, was getting agreement to allow nurses into college membership, which was eventually achieved. Since then, and with collaboration from the Royal College of Nursing, the formal standards and procedures for those practicing Travel Medicine have been defined. following this I was honoured to receive an MBE for services to travel medicine, which I considered to be on behalf of our whole team.

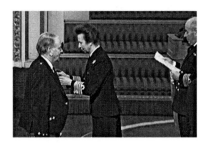

Global Health

Giving travel health advice involves assessing risks but also requires reliable, evidence based and continually updated information about global and regional disease patterns - a challenging task. Many using this information when counselling travellers, understandably don't realise the amount of work involved. Collating this information requires close collaboration between those identifying risks, and those responding to disease outbreaks in every part of the world.

Like travel medicine, 'global health' is a relatively new discipline (from around the 1980s) that has responded to the concept and challenges of the 'global village'. It differs from 'world' or 'public' health which studies risks at a population level and 'international' health which focuses on distribution of resources between countries - 'inter-national'.

Perhaps because of my background interests in agriculture and environmental issues, I have found it very easy to see links between travel, the environment and human health. The global free-market has only taken off in a big way since the mid-1900s. Societies and communities have been radically changed as a result, making many dependent upon far away sources for essential goods: including food. Profit seeking and self-interest has lead to previously sustainable communities declining: unemployment, migration to cites and a lack of appreciation of our dependency upon a healthy environment for food production. All this has been made possible by the speed, ease and availability of international air and sea travel and transport; which in itself contributes to pollution, waste, global warming and climate change. In many societies there is no word for 'waste'. I will discuss this further in the second part of this book.

While discussions about the meaning of 'global health' could make up a book in itself, my understanding is that it takes, as its starting point, that health and disease should be studied from a global perspective. This should be embarked upon sensitively: with respect for different cultures, concepts of health, and the many differing ways people live. It is worth reflecting that dying children and the elderly can be seen as healthy despite having life threatening diseases. Ideally, this concept of global health takes into account human transience on earth and breaks from the commonly broadcast notion that financial assets, an ever increasing gross domestic product and a consumer society are the only ways health and happiness can be achieved. Global health acknowledges environmental and ecological factors influencing health. As such, it recognises that short term profit-driven gains can be at the expense of our environment and eventually our own health. Perhaps the underlying problem lies with the name given to healthcare in the UK in the 1950s: 'The National Health Service' instead of a more appropriate title 'The National Disease Service'.

I am not fond of the expression 'think globally, act locally'. Unless we isolate ourselves from modern means of communication, we have no choice now but to think globally. It is possible to participate in global issues beyond simply feeling pity and sympathy when watching the world on television. We need active involvement informed by empathy, love and compassion; by working with others towards a better and more equitable world for all.

At the same time remembering that cultural differences in lifestyles and behaviour are important and can have a sound and healthy basis - 'there are many different ways to make good bread'!

While bearing these factors in mind, we may choose to get involved ourselves through real life experiences. Those of us teaching and supporting young medical students, for example, quickly become very aware of how carefully planned elective periods of learning abroad can be eye-opening and life-changing. Our attitudes to how we behave towards others at home and how we care for our local environment are also frequently changed by genuine and compassionate overseas experiences.

The Interdependence
of Global Health and Travel Medicine

Giving travel health advice without thinking in global health terms may seem like eating apples without recognising that they come from trees, and that someone has to organise the harvesting, collection and distribution. Similarly, studying global health requires an understanding of the role travel, migration and displacement play in the spread of diseases.

Overland and sea travel used to be how infections were spread internationally, but now we also have very fast air travel. AIDS would almost certainly have remained a zoonotic disease confined to Central Africa if the human immunodeficiency virus had not spread worldwide through air travel since 1970s. Influenzal pandemics now take months rather than years to spread worldwide. Another way of seeing the link is to consider that if malaria was eradicated in Africa, this would save millions of African lives and at the same time protect travellers.

There are many other ways the two subjects are interlinked such as the impact of travellers on those living within the host countries; the health needs of migrants, asylum seekers and displaced persons; faster transport leading to international food trading where the interests of the receiving countries frequently take priority over the producers linked. Food security is a big issue when food is not produced and consumed locally, and this often leads to a lack of respect and appreciation of what goes into food production and results in a lot of wastage. The challenge seems to be convincing others that there are alternatives to profit orientated commercial and multinational food production, although it seems unlikely the tide will be turned in any major way. Yet small is beautiful ... !

The Future

Undergraduates have led the way recognising the importance of the global health approach, perhaps being less cluttered by preconceived and organisationally established notions of how things should be done. The student organisation Medical Students International (MEDSIN) has 36 branches in universities throughout the UK and its vision is 'A fair and just world, in which equity in health is a reality for all'.

It has been very en-
couraging to see the British
Travel Health Association enthusiastically also embrace
this concept and adjust its
name and mission to become
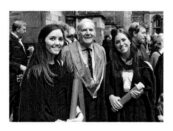
the British Global and Travel Health Association. Also
the British General Medical Council, in 2012, advised all
medical schools to include Global Health in their medical
undergraduate curriculum. This has already happened in all
the Scottish universities and increasingly in other parts of
the UK. The picture is of two of our first BSc in Global
Health medical students receiving their degrees in Glasgow.

It is interesting and understandable that general
practice seems to be the established specialty that has enthusiastically embraced global and travel health as a subspe-
cialty. In my experience, general practice is flexible when
it comes to taking on new initiatives and practitioners
often have the opportunity to take up part-time posts and
even sabbatical years. Sabbaticals can be taken abroad in
developing countries, supporting global health projects and
initiatives while undertaking voluntary work.

Since retiring from clinical practice I have helped
establish courses for medical students in Glasgow on
Global and Travel Health. There has been no shortage of
interest both for short 5 week intensive study modules and
for a 1 year intercalated Bachelors Degree course they can
undertake after their 3rd year of medical studies. Students
choose these courses as special subjects of interest to them,

so it is not surprising that they are constantly enthusiastic and committed to studying and learning about health from a global perspective. A frequent comment they make is that nowhere else in their undergraduate course are they introduced to basic concepts such as what we mean by the terms 'health', 'disease' and 'science'? We share both mine and their experiences, since many already have travelled abroad and may have undertaken gap years or volunteer work overseas. It is very rewarding to hear them describe the global health courses as inspiring, and I frequently can see reflections of my own 'journey' in their experiences through their questioning, critical appraisals and our discussions. They are only just starting on their journey as doctors and there will be many different ways and opportunities for them to develop these interests although they may need to recognise that some of their professional colleagues will see them as untraditional, unconventional and maybe even eccentric!

Four house moves were involved in this period, although all these were within the same Stirling district and for different reasons. Twenty years was spent in rented properties: a bungalow in Drymen and then a 'run-down' but beautiful very old farmhouse nearby. It was a great place for children to grow up in but had a lot of problems such as damp, and it was difficult to heat since we had to rely on wood-stoves strategically placed in the kitchen and in the living room (under the bedrooms). We were turned out of the farmhouse after 12 years when the farmer wanted to renovate it, and we moved into a small bungalow, again this time in Balfron, which was convenient for our children's schooling. Later we moved to an old estate manager's house near Aberfoyle which had the attraction of having more than 2 acres of land; including a paddock, small forested area and large natural pond.

This allowed scope for developing and experimenting with different ways of natural gardening. Regular guests (or maybe we were the guests) in the garden hosted a very wide variety of birds including a rookery and an occasional osprey as well as frogs, voles, toads and deer. Although many rabbits were in the area, few visited us (for which we were very grateful - see chapter, Work on the Farm Integrated with Nature) since the house was built on a raised rocky area surrounded by a flood plain of the Forth River. Rabbits seemed to have more sense than to try creating burrows in the lower fertile parts of our land where they would be flooded out several times a year. For similar reasons, we had no moles. I have now kept bees for more than 30 years.

I have also been involved in setting up a local reusing/recycling very successful charity shop 'Good Green Fun' which helps minimise the huge waste of children's clothes, toys, books, prams, games, cots etc. which so often are stored unused in attics, under beds or end up in landfill sites.

During the more settled time working in and living near Glasgow since the 1970s, many of my interests

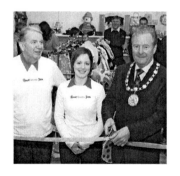

described previously were continued and developed further. These described here and others will be expanded upon in Part 2 of this book. It will include reflections on how rapidly, sometimes dramatically, our lives have changed due to our new ways communicating (through travel and technology). Also reflections on our relationship (or lack of) with the natural world, upon which we are dependent, and the impact these changes have on our health and our environment.

BIBLIOGRAPHY

*Just a few books relevant to the chapters
or ones I particularly remember*

The Children of the New Forest: Captain Marryat. Dean and Son Ltd (prior to ISBN) - (an adventure story about a family caught up in the revolution at the time of Charles I)

Small is Beautiful: E. F. Schumacher. 1974. Sphere Books. Then published by Vintage 2011 - (A classic and prophetic book on the impact of the consumer society on our environment)

Island Years, Island Farm: Fraser Darling. 1944 and following - recent reprint 2011. Little Toller Books. ISBN: 190 821 301 3 - (redeveloping a Scottish Island that had become uninhabited after the decline of the local fishing industry)

Scouting for Boys: Baden-Powell. 29th edition 1955. Pearson Press. (prior to ISBN) - (full of practical ways of camping and survival based on experiences in Southern Africa)

Swallows ands Amazons: Arthur Ransom. 1958. Lowe and Brydone. 0 224 60631 x - (the first of a series of childhood adventure stories emphasizing responsibility, self-reliance and initiative when facing difficulties)

Watership Down: Richard Adams. 1972 and following. Puffin Books - (basically a story demonstrating the power of love over evil)

St. Francis of Assisi - his life and writings: Leo Shirley Price. Mowbray Press. 1959 (prior to ISBN) - (we are a part of the whole of God's creation and we ignore this at our peril)

Les Miserables: Victor Hugo. 1909. 2 volumes. Dent & Sons Ltd. (prior to ISBN) - (a novel based about conversion, love, adventure and philosophy around the time of the French revolution)

The Christmas Mystery: Josrein Gaarder (also author of Sophie's World). 1992. Published in English 1996 by Phoenix House. ISBN 1 86159 015 6 - (A Norwegian classic - a moving journey of advent seen through the eyes of a young girl)

Clinical Methods: Robert Hutchinson 1897 (many later editions and reprints with additional contributors). Bailliere, Tindall and Cassell. ISBN 0 7020 0267 4 - (focuses on signs and symptoms so very relevant for work in countries where investigations are at a minimum)

A Primer of Medicine: M.H Pappworth 1960 and following. Butterworth & Co. ISBN 0 407 62601 8 - (focuses on signs and symptoms so very relevant for work in countries where investigations are at a minimum)

Medicine and Custom in Africa: Michael Gelfand. 1964. E & S Livingstone - (many informed observations on African culture at the time)

The Tissues of the Body: Le Gros Clarke. 1939 and following. ASIN: B001OVGLYS - (classic book about human anatomy and so readable it needs a mention)

Prayers: Michel Quoist. 1954 and following. Sheed and Ward ISBN 978 0 934134-46-0 (one of several his books focusing on the fundamental importance of fostering loving relationships with others)

The Donkey Walk: James Richards. 1967. Icon Books (prior to ISBN) - (love in old age)

Practicing Mindfulness: An introduction to meditation: Mark Muesse. 2011. Transcript of a 'Great Courses' audio download. ASIN: B00GGXK3IE - (a very readable introduction to this important subject which is coming into its own as a way of dealing with the stresses of a highly fast paced, technical and computer dependent world)

Natures Medicines: Richard Lucas. 1966 Award Books. ASIN: B000O86E7Q - (an informed and very readable treatise on the role of plants in medicine)

The No.1 Ladies Detective Agency: Alexander McCall Smith. 1998. Abacus Books ISBN 0 349 11675 X - (one of a series of novels giving an insight into African culture based on experience in Botswana)

Lightning Source UK Ltd.
Milton Keynes UK
UKOW02f2306250516

274999UK00001B/13/P